Pre-Hospital
Anesthesia Handbook

Andrew Griffiths
Tim Lowes
Jeremy Henning

Pre-Hospital
Anesthesia Handbook

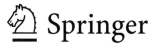 Springer

Lt Col Andrew Griffiths, MBBS
BMed Sci FRCA RAMC
Consultant in Anaesthesia
16 Close Support Medical
Regiment/ James Cook
University Hospital/GNAAS UK

Lt Col Tim Lowes, MBBS
FRCA Dip IMC.RCS(Ed) RAMC
Consultant in Anaesthesia & ICU
16 Close Support Medical
Regiment/ James Cook
University Hospital/GNAAS UK

Lt Col Jeremy Henning, MBBS
FRCA RAMC
Consultant in Anaesthesia & ICU
Ministry of Defence Hospital
Unit Northallerton/ James Cook
University Hospital
Clinical Director Great North
Air Ambulance Service UK

ISBN: 978-1-84996-158-5   e-ISBN: 978-1-84996-159-2

DOI 10.1007/978-1-84996-159-2

Springer London Dordrecht Heidelberg New York

British Library Cataloguing in Publication Data

A catalogue record for this book is available from the British Library

Library of Congress Control Number: 2010928390

Cover design: eStudioCalamar, Figueres/Berlin

Printed on acid-free paper

Springer is part of Springer Science+Business Media
(www.springer.com)

Foreword

The dramatic changes in the management of critically ill or injured patients in the pre-hospital environment that follow the implementation of lessons learnt in austere distant zones precede the publication of focused, evidence-based guides and manuals. This manual is therefore a great step forwards in training and assessment.

The commitment expressed in the Darzi report (High Quality Care for All – NHS Next Stage Review Final Report 2008) to provide the best care for all patients does mean that there will be occasions when primary resuscitation of patients is followed by a more prolonged transfer to definitive care. The opportunities to start and continue critical care of seriously ill patients by skilled anesthetists should provide the same benefits for civilian populations as has been demonstrated in hostile operations; a clear message from the Healthcare Commission (2009).

The authors are all experts in both the practical clinical application and the academic and research aspects of pre-hospital care. This manual covers the most important aspects of anesthesia and rightly concentrates on the safe and rapid establishment of a secure airway as part of the ongoing care of the patient. The techniques for rapid sequence induction of anesthesia are discussed and just as importantly so are the necessary subsequent anesthesia and sedation techniques.

This manual should be essential reading for all involved in the pre-hospital arena from paramedical to medical staff. It is a model for others to follow and it is a privilege to be asked to write this foreword.

Prof. Chris Dodds
JCUH

Preface

Over the past few years in the United Kingdom there have been many reports into trauma which have highlighted poor pre-hospital care as a major cause of possibly preventable deaths. Similar issues have been identified internationally. Many pre-hospital systems have therefore developed standard operating procedures that involve inducing anesthesia for airway control.

Many physician providers find it difficult to access training in this area, and assisting anesthesia is outside most paramedics' curriculum. This was a problem we faced at the Great North Air Ambulance Service. To address this, we developed a two day course to provide an introduction to pre-hospital anesthetic practice. This book has evolved from the manual we wrote for the course, which we continue to run three times a year.

It is clear that pre-hospital anesthesia remains a controversial procedure, with many conflicting papers written about its benefits and risks. For this reason, anyone undertaking it has a duty to ensure they undertake it safely and within a well governed system. A book cannot provide clinical experience, however, we hope that it will give a good knowledge-base to guide and develop practice. The available evidence is discussed, relevant pharmacology is explained and a system to provide pre-hospital anesthesia is presented.

We hope this book will prove to be an enjoyable read that will encourage many to develop their pre-hospital anesthetic practice. It has to be the hope of all working in this world that no patient ever dies from having inadequate airway control before their admission to hospital.

The authors acknowledge the support that the Great North Air Ambulance Service has given in the evolution of the course, and are donating all of their royalties from the sales of this book to the charity fund.

Middlesbrough, UK

Andy Griffiths
Tim Lowes
Jeremy Henning

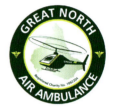

Contents

Aims and Objectives

- To be aware of the risks and benefits of Pre-hospital Anesthesia (PHA)
- To be familiar with the equipment and monitoring required to safely undertake Pre-hospital Rapid Sequence Intubation (PRSI)
- To increase competence at managing PRSI, including failed intubation
- To develop a comprehensive knowledge of the pharmacology of all PHA drugs, including indications, contraindications, doses and side effects
- To gain confidence in the preparation and transfer of the intubated patient and management of potential adverse events during transfer

Note: This handbook assumes experience with intubation, simple airway manoeuvres, bag-valve-mask ventilation and Advanced Life Support/Advanced Trauma Life Support protocols.

Chapter 1
Introduction

By the end of this chapter you will be able to:

- Define the term "rapid sequence intubation"
- Discuss the evidence regarding who should perform rapid sequence intubation
- Understand the challenges of pre-hospital rapid sequence intubation
- Discuss the evidence for and against pre-hospital intubation

1.1 Pre-Hospital Anesthesia (PHA)

The vast majority of general anesthetics undertaken in the pre-hospital environment will be commenced with a rapid sequence intubation (RSI). For this reason the majority of this handbook delivers the evidence, indications, contraindications, preparation for and performance of a pre-hospital RSI (PRSI). This technique is then supported by the equally important subject of post-intubation management, including the management and prevention of adverse events during transfer. Other techniques usually classed under the remit of anesthesia, including sedation and analgesia will also be covered, but the main focus remains PRSI.

A. Griffiths et al., *Pre-Hospital Anaesthesia Handbook*,
DOI: 10.1007/978-1-84996-159-2_1,
© Springer-Verlag London Limited 2010

1.2 Rapid Sequence Intubation

Rapid sequence induction is an anesthetic technique used to promptly induce anesthesia and optimize the conditions suitable for intubation in as short a time as possible (Box 1.1). Rapid sequence induction is therefore synonymous with rapid sequence intubation. It is usually undertaken in order to protect the airway from soiling by either oral (e.g., blood) or stomach contents, and is combined with the application of cricoid pressure. Although it was first described as a sequence of 15 steps by Stept and Safar (1970), Sellick's landmark publication on cricoid pressure in 1961 (Sellick 1961) alluded to the benefits of preoxygenation, intravenous barbiturate and a short-acting muscle relaxant as the ideal technique when there was risk of regurgitation on induction. RSI mitigates for the requirement to ventilate with a face-mask (and the associated risks of gastric insufflation and subsequent regurgitation that this entails) prior to intubation. The primary aim of RSI was to improve the safety of anesthesia for emergency surgery, where the risk of aspiration is highest. This technique remains extant, if not universal, in contemporary practice.

RSI is also utilized in the management of critically ill patients who have acute lung injury or bronchospasm, where mask ventilation may be insufficient to generate the

Box 1.1 The aim of the RSI

- Rapidly induce anesthesia[a]
- Rapidly achieve complete muscle relaxation to provide optimum intubating conditions
- Prevent airway soiling

[a]In unconscious patients, the aim of the induction agent is to attenuate the physiological response to intubation (i.e., hypertension, tachycardia and raised intracranial pressure).

necessary pressures to maintain adequate oxygenation. Prompt intubation should minimize the period of potential hypoxia by immediately providing the ability to achieve increased airway pressures and positive end expiratory pressure (PEEP).

There are several recipes used to achieve RSI, but all employ a combination of:

- A sedative agent to provide amnesia and obtund the response to intubation e.g., etomidate
- A neuromuscular blocking agent to provide paralysis and optimum intubating conditions e.g., suxamethonium

1.2.1 Who Should Perform RSI?

RSI is undertaken successfully by clinicians other than anesthetists and is now considered an essential part of emergency medicine training (FCEM curriculum version 3 – April 2006). Whether emergency department (ED) staff should be performing RSI unsupervised by an anesthetist as *routine* practice is debatable.

The conduct of RSI outside of an operating theater is associated with a higher rate of poor views at laryngoscopy and increased complication rates (Taryle et al. 1979). It can be reasonably assumed that these differences are related to the familiarity of theater staff to their equipment and environment. This is generally not the case elsewhere in the hospital or in the prehospital environment. This problem is compounded by the fact that the sub-set of patients requiring emergency airway interventions outside theater tend to be more physiologically compromised, have a higher requirement for manual in-line stabilization (MILS) and are generally more complex to manage.

The two largest UK studies of ED RSI comparing ED staff to anesthetists suggested that anesthetists achieved significantly better views at laryngoscopy and had a greater success rate for first-pass intubations (Graham et al. 2003; Stevenson et al. 2007). Another study, focusing on RSIs performed by critical care staff, reported a significantly higher incidence of multiple attempts and unsuccessful intubation by the first intubator (Reid et al. 2004). A large US study reinforces the significance of a well executed RSI by suggesting that the incidence of complications increases significantly when more than one attempt at intubation is required (Thomas 2004). Graham et al. reported almost 3 times as many esophageal intubations (17 vs. 6), twice as many episodes of severe hypotension (17 vs. 8) and twice as many endobronchial intubations (6 vs. 3) during ED staff RSI. Although the numbers overall were small, when RSIs at the main contributing center (Edinburgh Royal Infirmary) were analyzed, this was clearly statistically significant. Reid's study showed a significantly higher incidence of multiple attempts and unsuccessful intubation when the initial intubator was not an anesthetist; however overall (albeit self-reported) complications were similar. Similarly the Stevenson paper reported overall comparable complication rates for ED vs. anesthetic RSI. One might speculate that the episodes of hypotension requiring treatment might have been significantly reduced for anesthetists had they used etomidate for the majority of patients rather than propofol or thiopentone (ED 72% etomidate vs. anes 19%). This is probably because the majority of anesthetists were SHOs with little or no experience of using etomidate, whereas the majority of ED physicians were consultants. Despite this, the anesthetists had no more episodes of hypotension than the ED staff. Familiarity with the side effects and appropriate doses of induction agents, and the ability to minimize and manage adverse effects is as important as the ability to get the tube in with the best view. It may be, therefore, more appropriate for a senior ED physician to perform RSI than a junior anesthetic trainee. However, in an ideal world, a middle or senior grade anesthetist would inevitably add value.

It is vital to recognize that specialities other than anesthetics will acquire and want to maintain their skills. It is essential that this be supported, while giving due regard for patient safety. This is the spirit of the joint RSI protocol in Edinburgh, in which a senior anesthetist or intensive care specialist provides immediate support whilst trained ED staff perform RSI. This initiative was developed after the original data was analyzed. This approach has reduced the complication rate for the emergency physicians in a follow up study.

1.3 Pre-Hospital Rapid Sequence Intubation (PRSI)

1.3.1 The Pre-Hospital Environment

The pre-hospital environment is one of the most challenging clinical settings in which to practice. It can be austere as well as emotionally and physically demanding. The conditions are at best suboptimal, characterized by difficult access to the patient, limited equipment, inclement weather conditions and poor lighting (too dark or too bright). All these facets and many other stressors can hinder the performance of an optimal PRSI. The pre-hospital practitioner is also largely unsupported in terms of additional medical assistance and specialist airway equipment in the event of difficulties. To compound matters, many patients will have sustained head or neck trauma, resulting in difficult intubating conditions even in the controlled environment of a hospital. Despite these issues, the threshold to intubate is often lower; influenced by both the mode of onward transport and predicted transfer times to definitive care.

1.3.2 The Evidence for PRSI

Anecdotal reports exist that PRSI has been practised since 1972. The first report in the literature of PRSI was in 1988 (Hedges et al. 1988). The technique has been adapted from hospital practice. Intubation and ventilation in hospital is often considered a cornerstone in the management of critically ill patients. The optimum timing for this intervention has never been studied but it is assumed that the earlier the intervention takes place the greater the benefit it will offer. It has not been proven that RSI in the emergency department (vs. theater or ICU) improves outcome and reduces mortality, and probably never will be, as it is now accepted practice. This may well become the case with PRSI and it is clearly possible that the risks of carrying out this procedure in the pre-hospital setting may not outweigh the benefits. In other words, when RSI is undertaken in suboptimal conditions there is the potential for increased morbidity and mortality. In the absence of evidence clearly showing the benefit of PRSI a conservative approach may be appropriate.

There is currently no randomized controlled data showing clear benefit in mortality or morbidity following pre-hospital intubation. The only randomized controlled trial of pre-hospital intubation performed so far involved paramedics intubating children without drugs (Gausche et al. 2000). In addition to the lack of doctors and drugs (i.e., not PRSI), the study had major flaws. There have been several retrospective studies conducted in this area, and overall these have not been conclusive. Some of the studies suggest survival advantage (Winchell and Hoyt 1997; Arbabi et al. 2004). Others showed no improvement in neurological outcome or mortality (Stockinger and McSwain 2004). Other studies appeared to show an adverse outcome from pre-hospital intubation (Murray 2000; Eckstein et al. 2000).

When critically analyzed, the published evidence does not show PRSI to be detrimental and, as part of a Helicopter Emergency Medical Service (HEMS), is very likely to be beneficial. The vast majority of studies were from the US (several from the same trauma database) and involved paramedics, several using either no drugs or simply sedation with midazolam and no neuromuscular blocking agent (NMDA). Both failed intubation and other complications are reduced by the use of NMDAs (Bulger et al. 2005). These trials, most of which suggest inferior outcomes, are therefore clearly not applicable to PRSI. The study by Davis et al. of paramedic PRSI in traumatic brain injury compared to historical controls was associated with an increase in mortality (Davis et al. 2003). Periods of reduced SpO_2, and hyperventilation were noted and the relatively limited training and experience of paramedics were cited as potentially important factors.

Services such as the Whatcom Medic One (Washington state) have a relatively small number of well-trained paramedics using a recognized PRSI technique and report very good results (Wang et al. 2004). It is perhaps not surprising that those with large numbers of paramedics with very limited training and only occasional RSI experience tended to show worse outcomes. Improved outcome has been demonstrated for patients transferred by helicopter compared to land ambulance (Davis et al. 2005). This may be due to speed of transfer to hospital, better trained staff or a combination of both. Together this leads to the conclusion that small teams of well-trained staff on board helicopters are likely to improve outcomes if they are able to perform PRSI in certain patients.

One way to respond to the studies available is to follow the principle of "Primum non nocere" (first, do no harm). It would seem reasonable to assume that the minimum input to achieve a patent airway and adequate ventilation should be recommended. This can be achieved, in some cases by simple airway maneuvers with or without the use of adjuncts and a bag-valve-mask. Although this does not confer any degree of airway protection, it may allow rapid transfer from the scene.

There is an alternative view endorsed by Great North Air Ambulance, London HEMS and an increasing number of other pre-hospital helicopter medical services in the UK. It is a view that is based on the principle that optimal critical care provision should be available for those patients who require it at the earliest opportunity. In hospital this would invariably include intubation and therefore PRSI is an essential part of HEMS training. Many helicopter systems worldwide also provide this capability as part of their service provision.

1.3.3 Who Should Perform PRSI?

The restrictions on UK paramedic practice means that one member of the team must be a doctor if PRSI is to be undertaken. This is supported by one paper from Australia that reported an increased rate of intervention and delivered a significantly reduced mortality when a doctor was included in the helicopter rescue team (Garner et al. 1999). Exactly what training that doctor should have is contentious and unclear.

Rapid sequence intubation is one of the most complex and involved procedures that can be performed in the pre-hospital environment (Box 1.2).

Ultimately it requires a degree of self-confidence and the belief that you can be successful. This must be tempered by a respect for the risks involved and the potential for worsening patient outcome. Given the potential for difficult intubating conditions, discussed above, and the in-hospital studies that show anesthetists achieve better laryngoscopic views and more first time intubations, it may appear that PRSI should ideally be performed by an anesthetist. The situation is not quite so straightforward however. It must be remembered that:

(a) There are several other parts to medical care in the pre-hospital environment that the average anesthetist would not be as familiar or competent with (although many of these could be managed by a supporting paramedic).
(b) Pre-hospital care practitioners in the UK have traditionally been either GPs or ED physicians and there are relatively few anesthetists who are comfortable and have the experience of working in this environment.

Currently a compromise is often made either one way or the other (i.e., GPs/ED physicians with minimal anesthetic experience or anesthetists with limited ED/pre-hospital experience). In the future, specific training in pre-hospital care should provide HEMS doctors with sufficient experience in all relevant areas, and importantly, continuing professional development to maintain knowledge and skills.

The Pre-hospital Anesthesia working party from the Association of Anesthetists of Great Britain and Ireland has produced guidelines which state "The Acute Care Common Stem (ACCS) program, or equivalent training, should be regarded as the absolute minimum training required by an individual practicing pre-hospital anesthesia. However, specific training for working in the pre-hospital environment is also essential. Closely supervised working by experienced practitioners is an essential step to independent pre-hospital practice. Assessment of competence in pre-hospital anesthesia should always involve direct pre-hospital observation by practicing senior clinicians" (AAGBI 2007). An ACCS program includes 6 months each of emergency medicine and acute medicine and 1 year in anesthesia and intensive care medicine. Whether doctors who do not fulfill these criteria but who already provide pre-hospital anesthesia should continue to do so is down to the experience and judgment of the individual concerned, along with those responsible for pre-hospital clinical governance in the local area.

The importance of training and experience does not apply solely to the physician undertaking PRSI. Anesthesia in hospital is conducted only in the presence of an appropriately trained assistant. The same standards should apply in pre-hospital care. Invariably the assistant is a HEMS paramedic. An experienced and well-trained paramedic can be invaluable, particularly in more difficult situations.

Box 1.2 Skills required for an effective PRSI

- Technical skills to complete over 100 specific steps
- Cognitive skills to assess patient status and the appropriateness of the intervention
- Judgment to decide the appropriate time to initiate the procedure
- Problem solving skills to trouble-shoot during episodes of patient deterioration

1.4 Confidential Enquiry into Peri-Operative Deaths (NCEPOD): Trauma – Who Cares?

The recent NCEPOD report in the UK entitled "Trauma – who cares?," clearly recognizes the current unsatisfactory state of pre-hospital airway management and advocates increasing the numbers of staff able to perform PRSI (NCEPOD 2007).

The principle recommendations of NCEPOD included the following: "There is a high incidence of patients arriving at hospital with a partially or completely obstructed airway. Change is urgently required to provide a system that reliably provides a clear airway with good oxygenation and control of ventilation. This may be through the provision of personnel with the ability to provide anesthesia and intubation in the pre-hospital phase...." This handbook provides a basic working knowledge, based on the experience of the authors as taught and practiced at the Great North Air Ambulance in the UK.

Summary

- The pre-hospital environment is the most challenging clinical setting in which to work.
- RSI is the most complex procedure performed in the pre-hospital environment.
- The practitioner should be experienced and trained both at performing RSI and working in the pre-hospital environment.

References

Pre-Hospital anaesthesia; Association anaesthetists Great Britain and Ireland (London) 2009

Arbabi S, Jurkovich GJ et al (2004) A comparison of pre-hospital and hospital data in trauma patients. J Trauma 56:1029–1032

Bulger EM et al (2005) The use of neuromuscular blocking agents to facilitate prehospital intubation does not impair outcome after traumatic brain injury. J Trauma 58:718–723

Davis DP et al (2003) The effect of paramedic rapid sequence intubation on outcome in patients with severe traumatic brain injury. J Trauma 54:444–453

Davis DP et al (2005) The impact of aeromedical response to patients with moderate to severe traumatic brain injury. Ann Emerg Med 46:115–122

Eckstein M, Chan L, Schneir A, Palmer R (2000) Effect of pre-hospital advanced trauma life support on outcomes of major trauma patients. J Trauma 48:643–648

FCEM curriculum version 3 – April 2006, Appendix 3

Garner A, Rashford S, Lee A, Bartolacci R (1999) Addition of physicians to paramedic helicopter services decreases blunt trauma mortality. Aust N Z J Surg 69:697–701

Gausche M, Lewis RJ, Stratton SJ (2000) Effect of out-of-hospital paediatric endotracheal intubation on survival and neurological outcome: a controlled clinical trial. JAMA 283:783–790

Graham CA et al (2003) Rapid sequence intubation in Scottish urban emergency departments. Emerg Med J 20:3–5

Hedges JR, Dronen SC, Feero S, Hawkins S, Syverud SA, Shultz B (1988) Succinyl-choline-assisted intubations in pre-hospital care. Ann Emerg Med 17:469–472

Murray JA (2000) Pre-hospital intubation in patients with severe head injury. J Trauma 49:1065–1070

NCEPOD (2007) Trauma: who cares? National Confidential Enquiry into Patient Outcome and Death, London

Reid C, Chan L, Tweeddale M (2004) The who, where, and what of rapid sequence intubation: prospective observational study of emergency RSI outside the operating theater. Emerg Med J 21:296–301

Sellick BA (1961) Cricoid pressure to control regurgitation of stomach contents during induction of anaesthesia. Lancet 2:404–405

Stept WJ, Safar P (1970) Rapid induction – intubation for prevention of gastric content aspiration. Anaes Analg 49:633–636

Stevenson AG et al (2007) Tracheal intubation in the emergency department: the Scottish district hospital perspective. Emerg Med J 24:394–397

Stockinger ZT, McSwain NE (2004) Pre-hospital tracheal intubation for trauma does not improve survival over bag-valve-mask ventilation in trauma patients. J Trauma 56:531–536

Taryle DA, Chandler JE, Good JT, Potts DE, Sahn SA (1979) Emergency room intubations-complications and survival. Chest 75:541–543

Thomas CM (2004) Emergency tracheal intubation: complications associated with repeated laryngoscopic attempts. Anaes Anal 99:607–613

Wang HE, Davis DP, Wayne MA, Delbridge T (2004) Prehospital rapid-sequence intubation-what does the evidence show? Prehosp Emerg Care 8:366–377

Winchell RJ, Hoyt DB (1997) Endotracheal intubation in the field improves survival in patients with severe head injury. Arch surg 132:592–597

Chapter 2
Indications and Decision Making

By the end of this chapter you will be able to:

- Assess the risks and benefits of pre-hospital rapid sequence intubation
- Discuss the significance of aspiration
- Determine the need for intubation

The decision to escalate airway management from basic to advanced is not always clear cut. The primary aim must always be to maintain reliable airway patency and ensure adequate oxygenation and ventilation in order to prevent hypoxia and hypercarbia. The airway is at risk from aspiration or soiling from upper airway debris if the laryngeal reflexes are incompetent or rendered ineffective by drugs. A simple approach may not be the most appropriate as it is labor intensive and unreliable. In these cases, or if clear indications exist, consideration should be given to endotracheal intubation (Boxes 2.1 and 2.2).

A. Griffiths et al., *Pre-Hospital Anaesthesia Handbook*, 13
DOI: 10.1007/978-1-84996-159-2_2,
© Springer-Verlag London Limited 2010

Box 2.1 Indications for PRSI

Airway problems that cannot be reliably managed by simple maneuvers e.g., severe facial injury.

Respiratory insufficiency (SpO_2 <92%) despite 15 L/min O_2 or impending respiratory collapse due to exhaustion or pathology.

Glasgow coma scale (GCS) rapidly falling or <9.

Patients at risk of respiratory deterioration when access is difficult during transfer to definitive care e.g., facial burns.

Patients requiring sedation prior to transfer to hospital because they present a danger to themselves or attending staff or for humanitarian reasons e.g., provide complete pain relief.

Box 2.2 Contraindications to PRSI

Known anaphylaxis to one of the drugs required for intubation (although there may be an alternative).

Obvious physical deformity making successful intubation unlikely.

Croup or epiglottitis.

Stridor due to upper airway swelling/edema e.g., burns (when rapid transfer to hospital is indicated; cricothyroidotomy is the safest technique if respiratory failure develops in a pre-hospital setting).

2.1 Significance of Aspiration

The significance of aspiration in the pre-hospital environment is unclear. The risk of aspiration is dependent on patient injury, the nature of the aspirate and the absence of effective airway reflexes. Patients with neurological injury are at particularly high risk. Death due to aspiration usually occurs in two ways: Massive or particulate aspirates lead to upper or lower airway obstruction and asphyxiation. Smaller volumes may cause pneumonia, pneumonitis and/or acute respiratory distress syndrome (ARDS).

2.1.1 Incidence, Morbidity and Mortality of Aspiration

The incidence of aspiration in non-survivors from trauma has been reported to be up to 54% (where aspiration was defined as the presence of blood, vomit or other material in the upper respiratory tract at post-mortem) (Yates 1977). Another study group consisting of both survivors and non-survivors had an overall aspiration rate of 6% (McNicholl 1994). Hence aspiration may be a major contributor to trauma deaths or simply a marker of injury severity and an indicator of poor outcome (i.e., these results may indicate that aspiration increases mortality or that severely injured patients, who are more likely to die, are more prone to aspiration). Ottosson (1985) and McNicholl (1994) demonstrated aspiration only in those patients with non-survivable injuries. Yates (1977) believed that only some of the *in*-hospital deaths secondary to airway obstruction/aspiration could have been avoided. Hussain reviewed 152 pre-hospital deaths and concluded that at least 60 patients who died before reaching hospital had injuries that they might have survived (Hussain and Redmond 1997). He concluded that up to 85% of those who died before reaching hospital and had injuries that they could have survived, may have died with airway obstruction, *however*, all deaths occurred before medical or paramedical help arrived. He therefore advocated knowledge of basic airway protection and the recovery position as part of the driving test (86% of deaths were due to road traffic collisions (RTCs).

Further to this, it was noted that aspiration had occurred in up to 27% of head injured patients with GCS <9 prior to the arrival of medical help (Vadeboncoeur et al. 2006). In another study, the incidence of aspiration of those intubated on scene compared with those intubated in the ED was shown to be significantly greater (50% vs. 22%) (Ufberg et al. 2005). As paramedics tend to only intubate those with significantly reduced GCS pre-hospital, this again suggests that those who are most at risk are likely to have aspirated by the time pre-hospital teams arrive.

It should now be appreciated that pre-hospital evidence to recommend intubation as a means to prevent aspiration and reduce mortality does not exist. Hospital data has therefore been extrapolated. Perioperative aspiration is associated with around 4% mortality (Kluger and Short 1999; Warmer et al. 1993). In addition, casualties who aspirate have a longer Intensive Care Unit stay and poorer neurological outcome (Bronchard et al. 2004) when compared with those that do not, despite comparable injuries. Given this information and the fact that patients with a GCS <8 on scene do survive with good outcomes, it would seem reasonable to try and prevent aspiration where possible. In addition it should be remembered that if aspiration causes death pre-hospital, the cause is hypoxia. If aspiration has already occurred, hypoxia may be improved by rapid airway management and supplemental oxygen but may require intubation and ventilation to achieve satisfactory oxygenation in some patients.

2.2 LMA vs. Endotracheal Tube

In patients who have evidence of airway soiling, the majority of debris originates from the mouth or nose, with a low incidence of soiling from gastric contents (McNicholl 1994; Lockey et al. 1999). This suggests that a laryngeal mask airway (LMA), that provides some protection from soiling from above, may provide reasonable protection in the majority. It should be remembered that the act of inserting an LMA without prior administration of drugs may provoke vomiting or regurgitation. As a rule if the level of consciousness has allowed the placement of an oropharyngeal airway, an LMA will usually be tolerated. An ETT may be required anyway if increased airway pressures and PEEP are necessary to maintain adequate oxygenation.

2.3 Summary

The question remains whether the risks of an unprotected airway and potential aspiration (or further aspiration) justify the unproven benefit of intubating a patient prior to admission to hospital. As most airway soiling is caused by blood, a simple airway with adequate suction may be sufficient. Adequate oxygenation and ventilation may, however, require an endotracheal tube. An endotracheal tube is the gold standard for airway protection, but the benefit pre-hospital has not been shown.

2.4 Assessment of Need: Risk vs. Benefit

When making an assessment of the requirement for intubation it is important to balance the benefits of the intervention against the risks of performing it (Boxes 2.3 and 2.4).

Box 2.3 Benefits of intubation

- Provides a secure airway
- Allows ventilation with no leak and avoids gastric distension
- Allows administration of high FiO_2 and PEEP
- Provides protection to lungs from soiling with gastric contents and blood
- Allows bronchial suctioning

Box 2.4 Risks of intubation

- May lead to loss of airway and cerebral injury or death.
- May be complicated by periods of hypoxia or hypercapnia.
- Esophageal intubation, if unrecognized will be fatal.
- Endobronchial intubation may result in deterioration rather than improvement in oxygenation.
- Trauma to the airway including teeth, pharynx, larynx, and trachea.
- Worsening of airway obstruction if intubation fails e.g., burns, epiglottitis.
- Exacerbation of spinal injury.
- Coughing and gagging leading to an increase in intra cranial pressure (ICP).
- Regurgitation or vomiting during the procedure increasing the risk of airway soiling.
- Cardio-vascular instability resulting from laryngoscopy or drug administration.
- Barotrauma due to the application of high airway pressures during ventilation resulting in pneumothorax or tensioning of a simple pneumothorax.

2.4.1 Factors to Consider (The A B C D Approach)

2.4.1.1 Airway

It can be difficult to assess if the airway reflexes are intact. The gag reflex may be absent in 37% of otherwise healthy people (Davies et al. 1995). Attempting to elicit the reflex may stimulate vomiting and is not recommended. Absence of pharyngeal sensation is a more specific test for risk of aspiration. The presence of swallowing and the ability to clear secretions from the upper airway is therefore a more useful sign and implies coordinated upper airway function. Conscious patients with oral blood from maxillo-facial trauma may be managed best simply by sitting them forward and escorting them to hospital (with cervical protection if indicated).

2.4.1.2 Breathing

Hypoxia may result from chest pathology or inadequate ventilation. A physical examination may reveal treatable causes and these should be immediately addressed (e.g., tension pneumothorax). The patient with a large open pneumothorax may entrain air through their wound rather than down their trachea whilst spontaneously breathing. These patients should be managed by applying a self adhesive one way valve (e.g., Asherman or Bolin) or occlusive dressing and chest drain. Intubation may then not be required. Improvements in oxygenation and ventilation can be achieved from the provision of analgesia or by altering the patients' position (uninjured side is uppermost). Sitting the patient up can also improve respiratory dynamics and can be useful for left ventricular failure.

2.4.1.3 Circulation

Intravenous access used to be a prerequisite for RSI, but adult intraosseous access devices are now available and can offer a reliable alternative to cannulation. Suitable sites include the sternum, humerus and tibia. PRSI has been safely performed using this approach.

Hypovolemic patients will become hypotensive after induction. A reduced dose of induction agent should be considered. Fluid bolus and/or vasopressors should be prepared and given as required. Immediate transfer to definitive care for early surgery without intubation may be indicated. This is particularly applicable to patients with blunt abdominal trauma, who can markedly decompensate after induction. This can result from the loss of abdominal tone and its tamponade effect. Severe hypotension and cardiac arrest can swiftly follow drug administration. Delaying RSI until the patient is in the operating theater with a surgeon ready to perform a laparotomy may be the best option.

2.4.1.4 Disability

A GCS of less than 9, or a progressive deterioration in the score, is a strong indication for intubation. Agitation or aggression may necessitate the need for sedation and intubation to safely transport a patient. It should be remembered, however, that intubation to make an otherwise stable patient suitable for air transfer is inappropriate if a ground vehicle is available and an appropriate receiving hospital is within a short traveling time.

In addition to assessing A, B, C, and D, the following points need consideration:

- The environment and its suitability for the intervention
- The team's expertise and available personnel (minimum of one assistant required)
- The distance to definitive care and the speed and means of transfer
- The availability of equipment (minimum monitoring standards are required)
- The significance of not intervening

A decision-making algorithm can be found in Appendix "Decision Making Algorithm."

Summary

- The priority in pre-hospital care is to ensure a patent airway and adequate ventilation.
- The risk and benefit should be considered prior to intubation for each patient.

References

Bronchard R, Albaladejo P, Brezac G, Geffroy A, Seine PF (2004) Early onset pneumonia: risk factors and consequences in head trauma patients. Anaesthesiology 100:234–239

Davies AE, Kidd D, Stone SP, MacMahon J (1995) Pharyngeal sensation and gag reflex in healthy subjects. Lancet 345:487–488

Hussain LM, Redmond AD (1997) Are pre-hospital deaths from accidental injury preventable? BMJ 79:226–240

Kluger MT, Short TG (1999) Aspiration during anaesthesia: a review of 133 cases from the Australian Anaesthetic Incident Monitoring study (AIMS). Anaesthesia 54:19–26

Lockey DJ, Coats T, Parr MJA (1999) Aspiration in severe trauma: a prospective study. Anaesthesia 54:1097–1098

McNicholl BP (1994) The golden hour and pre-hospital care. Injury 25:251–254

Ottosson A (1985) Aspiration and obstructed airways as the cause of death in 158 consecutive traffic fatalities. J Trauma 25:538–540

Ufberg JW, Bushra JS, Karras DJ, Satz WA, Kueppers F (2005) Aspiration of gastric contents: association with prehospital intubation. Am J Emerg Med 23:379–382

Vadeboncoeur TF et al (2006) The ability of paramedics to predict aspiration in patients undergoing prehospital rapid sequence intubation. J Emerg Med 30:131–136

Warmer MA, Warmer ME, Weber JG (1993) Clinical significance of pulmonary aspiration during the perioperative period. Anaesthesiology 78:56–62

Yates DW (1977) Airway patency in fatal accidents. Br Med J 2:1249–1251

Chapter 3
Pre-Hospital Rapid Sequence Intubation

By the end of this chapter you will be able to:

- List the six P's of PRSI
- Discuss each of the P's in turn
- Appreciate the importance of a plan B

3.1 The Six P's

PRSI can be separated into six phases:

1. Preoxygenation
2. Preparation
3. Premedication
4. Paralysis and Sedation
5. Passage of the Endotracheal tube
6. Post intubation care

It is important that each member of the team is familiar with all phases of the RSI. This allows preparation to take place concurrently with ongoing patient management (Fig. 3.1).

A. Griffiths et al., *Pre-Hospital Anaesthesia Handbook*,
DOI: 10.1007/978-1-84996-159-2_3,
© Springer-Verlag London Limited 2010

"THE SIX P's"

PREOXYGENATION
5 min to GO

| High flow O_2 with reservoir mask |
| If SpO_2 < 90% provide PPV with BVM |
| *(and apply cricoid pressure)* |

PREPARATION
5 min to GO

| Preassessment (ABCDE) |
| Prepare equipment and drugs (PRSI checklist) |
| Position patient and team |
| Protect (c-spine & cricoid pressure) |

PREMEDICATION
2 min to GO

| Isolated head injury – Fentanyl |
| Paeds-? Atropine |

PARALYZE
(and sedate)
GO

| Induction |
| Cricoid pressure |

PASSAGE OF THE
ENDOTRACHEAL TUBE
30–45 sec from GO

| Use a Bougie |
| Locate cords and place ETT |
| Consider BURP or ease crioid pressure |
| Failed Intubation? |

POST INTUBATION CARE
1 minute from GO

| Inflate cuff |
| Confirm placement (capnography) |
| Cricoid pressure off |
| Secure tube |
| Check obs (BP/pulse) |
| Continue sedation+paralysis |
| ABCDEF Pre-transfer check |
| Transfer to hospital |

FIGURE 3.1. The 6 P's.

3.2 Preoxygenation

This is an essential phase. It provides a safety margin to prevent desaturation occurring in the period of apnoea prior to and during laryngoscopy. It should be performed using a tight

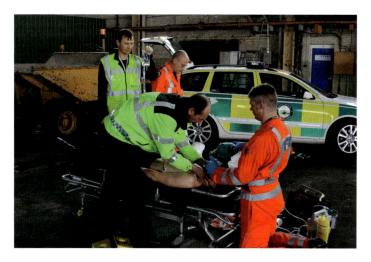

FIGURE 3.2. Preoxygenation being performed via a BVM with MILS being carried out.

fitting facemask with reservoir, preferably Bag-Valve Mask (BVM), for 3 min using 15 L/min of oxygen (Fig. 3.2).

In agitated patients it may be necessary to use sedation to facilitate pre-oxygenation. Small doses (1–2 mg) of midazolam should be titrated to affect. Patients who are hypovolemic and hypotensive may tolerate even these doses poorly. Ketamine (20–30 mg), titrated to affect, can be used in these patients but it is relatively contraindicated in head injury as it increases cerebral metabolic rate.

It may be necessary to augment the patient's own respiratory effort in order to maintain a SpO_2 above 94%, however, assisting ventilation may inflate the stomach and increase the risk of aspiration. Cricoid pressure will help to avoid this but may make ventilation more difficult in some cases.

The aim of preoxygenation is to replace the air in the functional residual capacity (30 mL/kg) of the lungs with an enriched oxygen mixture that will act as a reservoir for the body during apnoea. In ideal conditions this offers several minutes before desaturation (Fig. 3.3, Box 3.1).

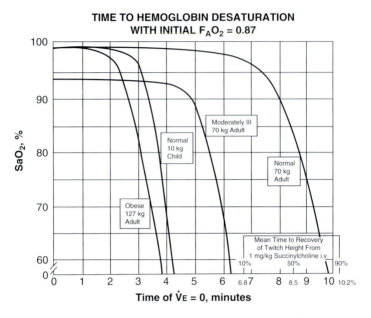

FIGURE 3.3. Desaturation curves after full pre-oxygenation.

Box 3.1 Time for desaturation to 90% after full preoxygenation (Benumof et al. 1997)

- 70 kg = 8.7 min
- 127 kg = <3 min (Pregnancy quicker)
- 10 kg = <4 min

3.3 Preparation

Performance of a rapid sequence intubation is not immediate and requires time for preparation. The time spent in the preparation phase is never wasted and will increase the chances of a swift and safe intubation. There are four elements to preparation for PRSI (Box 3.2).

Box 3.2 Preparation

- Preassessment
- Prepare equipment and drugs
- Position patient and team
- Protect (c-spine and cricoid pressure)

3.3.1 Preassessment

Preassessment should be easily remembered with a familiar ABCDE approach. It is a similar, but much more rapid assessment, to that which occurs before any anesthetic in the hospital environment.

3.3.1.1 Airway

The main concern is to achieve maximum patency to allow preoxygenation prior to PRSI. It is also useful to be able to predict the likelihood of "Difficult Airway."

3.3.1.2 Difficult Airway

The definition of a difficult airway is that a trained clinician experiences difficulties with mask ventilation, endotracheal intubation or both. Difficult mask ventilation is defined as a situation when it is impossible to maintain SpO_2 above 90% or it is not possible to reverse signs of inadequate ventilation with a BVM and 100% oxygen (Practical guidelines for management of the difficult airway 1993). The incidence of difficulty in airway maintenance in trauma patients can be up to 18% (Smith and Dejoy 2001). The incidence of a difficult airway is likely to be higher in the pre-hospital environment, for reasons mentioned earlier. Airway assessment should therefore include a judgment of the likely ease of airway maintenance with a bag-valve mask as well as the potential for difficult intubation. The anticipation of difficulty may require a change of the initial management plan (Box 3.3).

Box 3.3 Reasons for difficulty in maintaining an airway

- Obesity
- The presence of a beard
- The edentulous patient
- Facial injury

3.3.1.3 Difficult Intubation

During assessment, it is important to make a judgment about the difficulty of intubation. Difficult intubation is defined as the requirement for an experienced laryngoscopist to take more than two attempts at using the same blade on direct laryngoscopy; be required to use an intubation adjunct or an alternative device after failed laryngoscopy (Practical guidelines for management of the difficult airway 1993). The Whatcom Medic One service reports a pre-hospital failed intubation rate of 3.4% (2,978 patients), although some intubated patients required three attempts (Wang et al. 2004). This is identical to the failure rate reported by Fakhry et al. (2006), again a paramedic service allowing up to three attempts at intubation (175 patients). In 1993 London HEMS, a physician led service, reported a requirement for surgical cricothyroidotomy in 7.7% of 143 patients requiring advanced airway management on scene (Xeropotamos et al. 1993). Since then PRSI training has been improved and the threshold for cricothyroidotomy increased. Recently they reported no failed intubations from 244 PRSIs performed over a 1 year period (Newton et al. 2008).

The Modified Mallampati classification of airway assessment (Fig. 3.4) is a commonly used tool in the hospital environment to predict difficult intubation but is often not possible in patients requiring PRSI. Other predictors of difficult intubation may be present (Box 3.4).

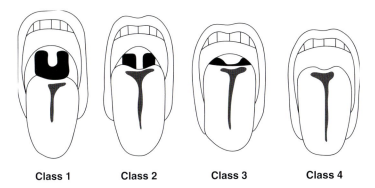

Class 1   Class 2   Class 3   Class 4

FIGURE 3.4. Airway assessment – Modified Mallampati classification. Reproduced by kind permission Anaesthesia UK Website.

Box 3.4 Reasons for difficult intubation

- Large upper incisors
- Limited mouth opening
- Reduced range of movement of the head/neck (MILS)
- Reduced sterno-mental distance ("no-neck"), thyro-mental distance ("chinless")
- Swollen/edematous tongue or laryngeal/pharyngeal tissue
- Congenital abnormalities
- Previous maxillo-facial surgery or radiotherapy

3.3.1.4 Clinical Signs of Potential Difficult Intubation or Ventilation

Obese Patients

Obese patients or those with short muscular necks can be difficult to intubate and ventilate. Excess soft tissue around the airway may hinder displacement during laryngoscopy. This may affect the view. These tissues may also collapse over laryngeal structures making manual ventilation difficult. Two-handed mask ventilation with a guedel may be required.

Edentulous Patients

Edentulous patients are often easy to intubate but can be difficult to manually ventilate. The teeth do not give support to the cheeks and as a result the face-mask seal may be poor. This can be remedied with a 2-handed technique bunching the facial tissue up into the mask to achieve a seal. Early intubation or use of an LMA may be required if ventilation is inadequate.

"Chinless" Patients

Patients with micrognathia (receding chin) usually have an anterior larynx. There is a reduced thyromental distance: tip of chin to thyroid cartilage (Adam's apple) of <6.5 cm *with the neck extended*. This measurement is therefore not practical when cervical spine injury is a concern. An impression of micrognathia should still be a visual clue. These patients do not have enough space to displace tissue forward to allow intubation. BURP and a bougie will often be required. (Note: Male patients often grow a beard to hide their anatomy.)

"No-Neck" Patients

The sternomental distance (tip of chin to sternum) is reduced (<12.5 cm) predicting a difficult intubation. Again, this measurement is based on the head in an extended position and is therefore not usually practical. Subjective appearance may add to your assessment of difficulty.

Bearded Patients

As well as sometimes hiding micrognathia, a beard makes it difficult to achieve an adequate seal with a facemask to allow ventilation. Applying lubricating jelly to the beard and using a two-person technique will improve the situation. An LMA may be required to ventilate if intubation is not possible.

"Goofy" Patients

A prominent overbite (protruding upper teeth) can impede laryngoscopy. It may be difficult to maneuver the laryngoscope without levering on the upper teeth. External pressure on the larynx (above the cricoid cartilage) and use of a Macintosh No. 3 blade, inserted fully inside the mouth (past the top teeth), may help.

"Stiff-Neck" Patients

In patients with poor neck mobility and no risk of neck instability, the larynx will, in effect, be more anterior. Elevating the head further to compensate for reduced extension of the head along with cricoid pressure and a bougie, gives the best chance of success. If there is a chance of underlying instability and risk of spinal cord injury (e.g., severe rheumatoid arthritis), no head or neck movement should take place. The only movement that is appropriate is jaw distraction.

Bleeding (Oral) Patients

Management of patients with blood in the oropharynx can present a particular challenge to the intubator. These patients are best managed in a slightly head-down position. This allows blood to pool in the upper pharynx away from the vocal cords. Adequate suction is the key to success; two suction devices may be required.

> Remember: A predicted difficult intubation may actually be easy but conversely some "easy" intubations turn out to be difficult. This necessitates the need for a fall back plan or "Plan B" (see text later).

3.3.1.5 Breathing

The initial assessment will have determined the urgency for PRSI. A hypoxic patient with a poor respiratory effort will prompt a more rapid response than one with adequate oxygenation and ventilation but who has a reduced GCS.

If a pneumothorax has been diagnosed, this should have been treated at least with needle thoracocentesis (Appendix "Needle Thoracocentesis") prior to intubation. Positive pressure ventilation can rapidly change a pneumothorax into a tension pneumothorax, resulting in profound cardiovascular collapse. A thoracostomy ± drain (Appendix "Thoracostomy ± Chest Drain Insertion") must be performed immediately after PRSI. (Note: Thoracostomy without a drain is only permissible in a *ventilated* patient. If the patient is breathing spontaneously, a thoracostomy will create an open pneumothorax, which will not improve ventilation. A valve system to prevent air entrainment during inspiration is therefore required i.e., a chest drain. (A needle/cannula thoracostomy is acceptable as this allows the release of a "tension" but is too small to allow any significant entrainment of air during inspiration)).

3.3.1.6 Circulation

Intravenous (IV) access must be gained (or checked with a 10 mL flush if already in place). This should then be *adequately secured* (IV sites are particularly vulnerable in the pre-hospital environment.) In the critically ill patient intraosseous (IO) access may be appropriate if two attempts at IV access have failed. Even in the pre hospital environment it is helpful to do this as aseptically as possible. 2% chlorhexidine in 70% alcohol wipes should be used to clean the skin, and minimal handling of the puncture site is advocated. Where this is not possible, it is worth noting that access was achieved in an emergency on the handover notes, so the receiving hospital can replace it as soon as practical.

The assessment of shock (inadequate tissue perfusion) in the pre-hospital patient can be difficult. Skin character and capillary return may be confusing in a cold environment. Confusion and level of consciousness may be lost as a guide to adequate perfusion if there is a coexisting head injury. Heart rate can be very useful, but is not specific to changes in volume status. Tachycardia may result from sympathetic stimulation secondary to inadequate analgesia (or sedation when the patient is intubated). Bradycardia may be due to beta-blockers, high spinal cord injury or be may be heralding a pre-terminal event.

In the absence of a measured blood pressure, the presence, site and character of peripheral pulses give useful information about cardiovascular status. It is suggested that the presence of a radial pulse implies a blood pressure of 80–90 mmHg and the presence of a carotid pulse equates to a blood pressure of 60–70 mmHg, although this has not been validated (Greaves et al. 2000). There is no doubt that the presence of a radial pulse implies a higher blood pressure than the presence of a carotid pulse alone.

When managing a profoundly hypotensive patient (i.e., no radial pulse palpable), the current consensus is to give a 250 mL fluid challenge (crystalloid) (Greaves et al. 2002). In the majority of pre-hospital cases, hypotension will be secondary to hypovolemia. If hemorrhage is external and easily compressible it may be reasonable to give further fluid to aim for a relatively normal Mean Arterial Pressure (MAP) for that patient. This is particularly appropriate if the patient has sustained a head injury and may have reduced Cerebral Perfusion Pressure secondary to a raised Intra cranial pressure (ICP). Conversely, if the hypovolemia is due to internal, non-compressible hemorrhage (diagnosed by transient or no response to a fluid challenge) current opinion is that further fluid should be withheld unless the radial pulse becomes impalpable once more. This is because these patients may actually be made worse by fluid resuscitation causing an increase in blood pressure and dislodgement of formed clot resulting in greater loss of blood. Consequently, the patient may be more coagulopathic and hypothermic on arrival to hospital and less likely to survive surgery. A compromise in target systolic pressure of 100 mmHg is recommended for patients with severe head injury *and* non-compressible hemorrhage. If the time to surgery is extended i.e., >1 hr the risk of renal failure and subsequent multi-organ failure becomes a real concern, and attempting to increase the blood pressure at this point may be the better option. Indeed the latest edition of the British Army's Battlefield Advanced Life Support (BATLS 2008) course, advocates "novel hybrid resuscitation," whereby hypotensive resuscitation is practiced for the first hour after injury, followed by normotensive resuscitation. The rational is that clot will form and become sufficiently robust in that first hour, to allow normal organ perfusion thereafter.

3.3.1.7 Disability

In head injury particular attention should be placed on pre-sedation pupil responses and GCS, particularly the motor score, as these have the most prognostic significance (along with age and CT scan appearance) (Murray et al. 2007). It should be documented and communicated on hand over. The presence of unilateral pupillary dilatation may be due to direct trauma or previous surgery, however, until proven otherwise it should be assumed to be a sign of raised intracranial pressure. The appearance of pupillary dilatation after initial normal appearance is particularly indicative of an expanding intracranial haematoma. Urgent transfer to a neurosurgical center for evacuation of haematoma is crucial. Mannitol or hypertonic saline should be given and temporary mild hyperventilation may be considered appropriate.

   Level of consciousness may also affect the amount of induction agent given, however it should be remembered that one of the reasons for giving the induction agent is to obtund the response to laryngoscopy. This dose may be similar whether the patient is unconscious or not.

3.3.1.8 Exposure

Exposure of the patient may have occurred to varying extents to allow a primary survey to be conducted. It is important to keep the patient protected from the elements where possible. The head and neck will clearly need to be exposed for intubation, as will the chest when confirming position afterwards.

Visualizing the larynx is likely to be more difficult in the presence of driving rain, sleet or snow, and unfortunately also in bright direct sunlight. It may be appropriate to move the casualty prior to attempting intubation in adverse weather conditions, e.g., undercover or into an ambulance. Alternatively a ground sheet or similar may be held above the casualty if other emergency service personnel are able to assist. (Note: In certain situations, access to intubate the patient may be severely restricted and in these cases it is invariably safer to move the casualty first.)

Inducing and paralyzing a patient in a confined area is asking for trouble. A nasopharyngeal airway and rapid extraction is more appropriate. If the casualty remains trapped in a confined space, a surgical cricothyroidotomy on a spontaneously breathing casualty with local anesthetic infiltration (if alert), is likely to be safer than attempting PRSI. It is also worth noting that in a CBRN (Chemical, Biological, Radiological, Nuclear) environment most authorities advocate simple airway maneuvers until the casualty has been removed from the hazard and decontaminated.

3.3.1.9 History

If possible some basic history should be sought with special reference to anesthesia. The AMPLE history is acceptable (Box 3.5). If the patient is conscious, their name, date of birth and next of kin details allow for more effective administration in hospital.

> ## Box 3.5   The AMPLE history
>
> - Allergies
> - Medications
> - Past Medical History
> - Last meal
> - Events leading to injury

3.3.2 Prepare Equipment and Drugs

The equipment required for intubation should have a standard configuration and everyone in the team should be familiar with it. It should be packed so that all items are easily accessible. Equipment bags based on the tool roll principle can be effective for this purpose. They open out into a predictable configuration with individual items held securely in place. These items can be easily checked and are immediately at hand but are less likely to be left behind when withdrawing from the scene. Alternatively a "kit dump" can be prepared on a clean folded drape or clinical waste bag. This has the advantage of being easily seen and avoided by other emergency service personnel.

3.3.2.1 Pre-RSI Checklist (Appendix "Pre-RSI Checklist")

All equipment should be checked immediately prior to induction. The team do this together, with one calling out the list and the other checking the kit (Fig. 3.5). Laryngoscope handles should have working batteries and there should be two blades with functioning bulbs. An appropriately sized endotracheal tube (ETT) should be prepared: check the cuff does not leak, then fully deflate and lubricate it. An ETT a size smaller than estimated should also be easily accessible in case of unexpected difficulties. In patients with stridor or suspected airway edema, an ETT 1–2 sizes smaller than normal should be prepared.

A gum elastic bougie must be available. This should be checked for cracks or signs of weakness prior to use. A 10 mL syringe is required for inflating the ETT cuff and either tape or tie prepared for securing the position once placement is confirmed.

Minimal monitoring standards should be used routinely (Pulse oximeter, NIBP, capnography and ECG). In certain circumstances this may not be possible. A pulse oximeter may not function if the patient is cold or peripherally shutdown and

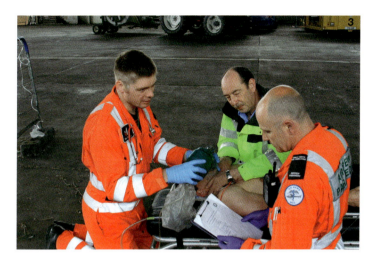

FIGURE 3.5. Challenge and response taking place using the checklist prior to induction.

even grossly assessing the color of the patient (blue vs. pink) may be difficult in poor lighting. NIBP may need to be done manually by palpation or simply by ensuring the presence of a radial pulse. $ETCO_2$ is the gold standard for confirming tracheal intubation and is also important for monitoring ventilation during transport, particularly in head injured patients (Figs. 3.6 and 3.7).

Sedative and paralyzing agents should be prepared in standard concentrations and carefully labeled using permanent ink on the syringe barrel. The doses are then calculated appropriately for the patient's weight and condition (Appendix "Drug Dose and ETT Size Field Card"). Drugs and doses should then be cross-checked with another team member. Preparing essential drugs on a daily basis or using commercial or pharmacy pre-filled syringes may be an option. This reduces the risk of dilution and labeling errors on scene. It also offers the advantage of a shorter preparation time.

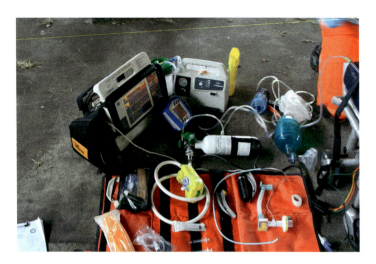

FIGURE 3.6. The equipment required to safely conduct a pre-hospital rapid sequence intubation.

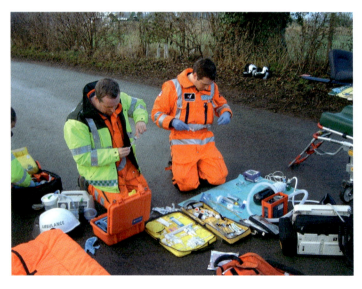

FIGURE 3.7. A trauma team drawing up drugs and preparing an equipment dump.

Daily prepared drugs can be wasteful and expensive though if their use is infrequent. It is important to remember that pre-filled suxamethonium syringes must still be refrigerated. Suxamethonium degrades over time and the rate of degra-dataion increases with higher temperatures.

3.3.3 Positioning

360° access to the patient is preferable during intubation and this should be ensured prior to induction in all cases where possible. In addition, it is usually easier to perform laryngos-copy with a patient off the ground. For this reason, if practi-cable, place the patient on a trolley or elevated spinal board prior to induction. Having the trolley at knee height with team members kneeling is ideal, as this allows equipment and monitors to be left on the ground but within reach.

The trained assistant is ideally positioned facing the intuba-tor on the side of the patient where IV access has been gained (it is slightly easier if this is on the patient's right so they can easily pass airway items into the right hand of the intubator, but makes little difference). The kit dump is placed between the intubator and assistant so that both are able to reach kit if required. If on the right side of the patient the assistant provides cricoid pressure with the right hand and passes equipment with the left and vice versa (Fig. 3.8). Given the potential for inap-propriately applied cricoid pressure to be either ineffective or to impede intubation, it is not advisable to ask others with little or no experience of the technique to take on this role.

If IV access is in the arm, either the intubator or the assis-tant should then be able to reach the cannula and administer drugs. It may be preferable (or necessary, e.g., tibial IO access) for another paramedic to administer drugs. In addi-tion this person can continuously palpate the radial pulse following induction to promptly detect the requirement for a vasopressor/inotrope/fluid. Instructions regarding drug doses must be explicit and understood prior to commencing PRSI.

The monitor is placed so that both the intubator and assis-tant can see it. This usually means next to the kit dump, but

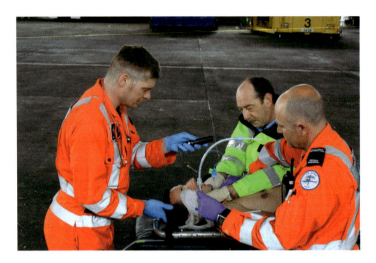

FIGURE 3.8. After induction a laryngoscopy is performed with cricoid pressure on and MILS if indicated from the history. If the ETT is mounted. If a bougie is used it increases the success rate of intubation at first attempt.

further away from the patient. If the patient is on a trolley, this may require the monitor to be tilted back to get a clear view of the screen. If manual in-line stabilization (MILS) of the cervical spine is required, it is carried out from the opposite side to the trained assistant. If any task is to be devolved it is MILS as it is relatively easy to instruct another member of the emergency services to undertake this role.

It may be useful to position a bystander at the foot of the casualty in order to tilt the patient head down should the oropharynx fill with vomit or blood during induction. A functioning high pressure, high volume suction unit should always be immediately to hand with a manual unit in reserve.

The "sniffing the morning air" position; with the neck flexed and head extended, is the ideal intubating position (Fig. 3.9), however this is not appropriate if there is a possibility of cervical spine injury.

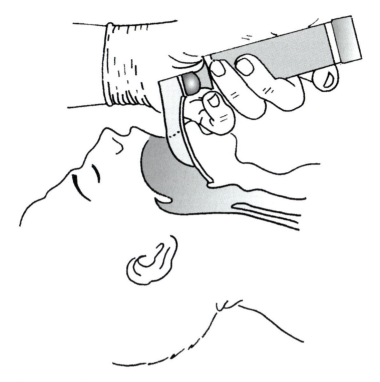

FIGURE 3.9. The performance of a laryngoscopy. Adapted from an image from www.anesthesiologists.org, with kind permission.

3.3.4 Protection

3.3.4.1 Cervical Spine Injury

2.4% of blunt trauma victims will have sustained a cervical spine injury. If the GCS is <8 this figure increases to 10.2% (Crosby 2006). The indications for PRSI (e.g., respiratory compromise, reduced GCS etc.), by definition, preclude pre-hospital clearance of the cervical spine. Therefore, if the mechanism of injury is consistent with a cervical spine injury, MILS should be initiated.

Manual In-Line Stabilization (MILS)

When three team members are present, MILS is best performed from the opposite site of the casualty to the assistant, approaching over the front of the chest (Fig. 3.10). MILS can be applied from above on either side of the intubator but this can impede the intubation process. The aim of MILS is to oppose the forces generated by laryngoscopy and is achieved by firmly holding down the patient's mastoid processes (Fig. 3.11). This affords a good mechanical advantage to oppose movement during laryngoscopy and reduces the degree of head extension by 50% (Hasting and Wood 1994). When only two team members are in attendance the intubator may have to improvise immobilization. This can be achieved by supporting the patients head between the thighs in a seated position with legs placed over either shoulder alongside the patients' chest. A "careful" intubation may be all that is possible.

If the patient is already immobilized with a hard collar and head blocks, these should be removed (the collar may simply be opened or the front part removed) and replaced by (MILS). Full spinal immobilization is independently associated with an increased risk of difficult intubation (Heath 1994). Removing the collar significantly improves mouth opening (Goutcher and Lochead 2005), but MILS will still impede a view at laryngoscopy compared to the optimum position. Nolan reported a reduced view in 45% of "normal" elective patients, with no view of the larynx at all in 22% (Nolan and Wilson 1993). Reassuringly, although five patients were unable to be intubated directly, all were intubated successfully with the use of a bougie. A bougie is superior to a malleable stylet to aid intubation (Gataure et al. 1996; Noguchi et al. 2003), and should be used routinely in PRSI to reduce the time to successful intubation. Performing a RSI with MILS using a gum elastic bougie is very unlikely to cause further cervical spine movement (Crosby 2006).

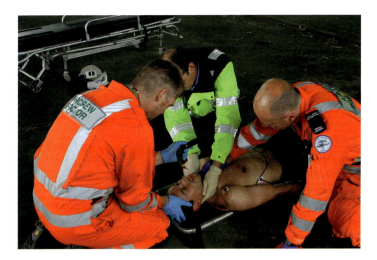

FIGURE 3.10. MILS can be performed over the chest from the opposite side to the assistant.

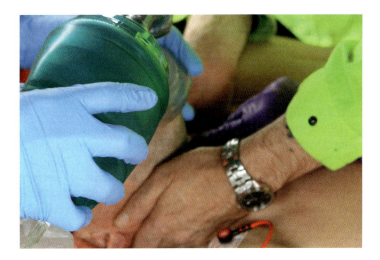

FIGURE 3.11. The aim of MILS is to fix the casualties head and neck during laryngoscopy to resist displacement and reduce the risk of cord injury to an unstable cervical spine.

Remember: Failure to oxygenate may kill the patient; moving the neck will probably not.

3.3.4.2 Cricoid Pressure

This is a technique used in anesthesia to decrease the risk of aspiration during induction. The application of cricoid pressure is also known as Sellick's maneuver after the anesthetist who first described it in 1961 (Sellick 1961). During induction the tone of the upper esophageal sphincter is reduced and the airway reflexes lost. This means that gastric contents may passively move up the esophagus, into the oropharynx and soil the airway. The application of cricoid pressure compensates for this loss of tone by compressing the proximal esophageal lumen between the cricoid cartilage and the cervical vertebrae.

The cricoid cartilage is chosen as it is the only part of the airway that consists of a complete ring of cartilage (Fig. 3.12). The thyroid cartilage and tracheal rings have only soft tissue posteriorly and are ineffective at compressing the esophagus.

Cricoid pressure is a 3-finger technique. Sellick described the maneuver as follows: "Before induction the cricoid is palpated and lightly held between the thumb and second finger; as anesthesia begins, pressure is exerted on the cricoid cartilage mainly by the index finger."

Sellick reported the technique as a 1-handed maneuver. Some groups have advocated the use of a 2-handed technique, with the second hand providing counterpressure behind the neck. This technique may have utility as when anterior force is applied, neck flexion is possible. This may potentially exacerbate a cervical spine injury. It appears, however, that when the correct force is used in the correct direction, there is no clear additional advantage to the provision of posterior neck support (Cook 1996; Vanner et al. 1997). Therefore, in both the hospital and pre-hospital environment a 1-handed technique is usual. This technique has the added advantage of allowing the assistant to deliver cricoid pressure and pass equipment during intubation.

Cricoid pressure should be applied as the patient loses consciousness or ceases respiratory effort (if already unconscious).

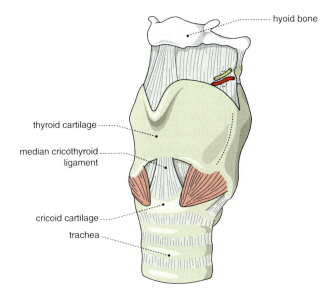

FIGURE 3.12. Upper airway anatomy.

It should not be released before the endotracheal tube has been placed, had the cuff inflated and its position confirmed. It is permissible to gently ventilate the lungs with cricoid pressure in situ, should it be necessary, to maintain the SpO_2 above 92% prior to laryngoscopy.

It has been shown that a force of 30 N is necessary to achieve esophageal occlusion and prevent regurgitation (Vanner and Asai 1999). This pressure is described as "firm pressure" or that required to cause pain when applied to the bridge of the nose.

More than 20 N of force is uncomfortable and can cause retching, so it is preferable to simply position the fingers over the cricoid cartilage prior to induction rather than apply excessive pressure too early.

Correctly applied cricoid pressure may enhance the laryngoscopic view and facilitate intubation in some patients. More likely, it will impede the view at laryngoscopy (Haslam et al. 2005). Excessive force (>40 N) may lead to distortion of the upper airway. This may make both intubation more difficult and impede mask ventilation in the event of a failed intubation. Cricoid pressure should be applied directly backwards, but it is easy to accidentally apply pressure to either the left or right (usually the opposite side to the person applying the pressure. The intubator should be aware of these potential problems and be prepared to move the hand of the assistant in an attempt to visualize the larynx. The intubator should have a low threshold for requesting reduction or even removal of cricoid pressure if they consider that their view is being impeded by its application.

In addition to the above problems, inadequate pressure may be ineffective and still allow regurgitation. Similarly pressure applied in the wrong place, e.g., thyroid cartilage, will not be effective either. Given the potential for problems, it is important that the assistant is trained and proficient in this technique, particularly when the intubator is relatively inexperienced. It is well recognized that even experienced anesthetic assistants may have a poor technique if not recently practiced. However, this can be easily improved by a very short period of simple retraining (Owen et al. 2002; May and Trethewy 2007). Experience in delivering the correct pressure can be achieved using mechanical simulators, infant or kitchen scales or even a 50 mL syringe (compressing the plunger on a capped off, air-filled 50 mL syringe to 33 mL approximates to 30 N) (Herman et al. 1996; Flucker et al. 2000).

If passive regurgitation occurs, pressure should be increased and the oropharynx suctioned immediately. Conversely, cricoid pressure should actually be released if active vomiting occurs at induction. This may occur before any/sufficient induction agent has been given and can sometimes be provoked by excessive and early cricoid pressure. In this case the continued application of force to the cricoid can result in esophageal rupture.

Given the evidence for pre-hospital aspiration described earlier, the benefit of cricoid pressure is not proven. It is most likely to be beneficial in those who have not yet lost laryngeal reflexes (i.e., GCS>8) but who will do so when an anesthetic is administered and may then be at risk of aspiration. To avoid confusion, it is advisable to utilize cricoid pressure for every PRSI, but to be aware of the limited evidence and have a low threshold for adjusting/releasing it when faced with a difficult intubation (Box 3.6).

> ## Box 3.6 Current recommendations for cricoid pressure (Smith and Dejoy 2001)
>
> - 10 N – Applied whilst conscious
> - 30 N – Applied with loss of consciousness

3.4 Premedication

Pretreatment with a drug (before giving the induction agent) is usually aimed at obtunding the sympathetic response to laryngoscopy whilst allowing a reduced dose of induction agent to be used to achieve the same end result. The pretreatment drugs are therefore ideally more cardiostable than the induction agents. Examples of drugs used for pretreatment include alfentanil and fentanyl.

3.5 Paralyze and Sedate

The induction phase should only be commenced when all preparation is complete. Other than in periarrest situations, the team should have already run through the Pre-RSI checklist to ensure that nothing has been missed.

PRSI should then begin with the administration of an induction agent (preceded by pretreatment if appropriate). The dose of the drug should be adjusted to account for level of consciousness, other drugs already given/taken, volume status, blood pressure and ICP. Most induction agents cause hypotension. This hypotension may result from peripheral vasodilatation, a reduction in cardiac contractility or a reduction in intrinsic sympathetic tone. Hypotension is most marked in hypovolemic patients but may not be immediately obvious after intubation due to the sympathetic response to laryngoscopy. Hypotension is a predictable side effect and vigilance with prompt management is essential. Ideally one attender should be tasked to monitor the radial pulse both during and after induction. Prophylactic treatment may be considered with a fluid bolus being administered prior to induction. A vasopressor or inotrope should be on hand to manage episodes of hypotension resistant to fluid therapy.

Loss of consciousness (e.g., loss of eyelash reflex or loss of verbal response) is normally assured prior to administration of the paralyzing (neuromuscular blocking) agent. Suxamethonium 1.5 mg/kg is traditionally used because of its rapid onset, but is associated with many side-effects (Box 3.7). However, there is still no other neuromuscular blocking agent (NMBA) that acts as rapidly as suxamethonium. It is frequently cited that a benefit of succinylcholine over other NMBAs is it short duration of action, in most cases. This means that in the event of failed intubation the patient re-commences spontaneous respiration and assist in oxygenation. In reality critical desaturation is likely to have occurred by this stage if the casualty has not been ventilated (Benumof et al. 1997). The "Failed Intubation Drill" should therefore always be initiated in the case of inability to intubate rather than waiting for the casualty to start breathing again.

The paralyzing agent should always be followed by a flush to ensure the drug reaches its point of action in as short a time as possible. The onset of paralysis usually takes place within 20–30 s, however in low cardiac output states this may be rather longer. When using suxamethonium its onset is usually heralded by fasciculations but these are not always seen. As a guide, laryngoscopy should be attempted only when the mouth opens freely. This equates well to cord paralysis.

Box 3.7 Side effects of suxamethonium

- Anaphylaxis
- Malignant hyperthermia (including masseter spasm)
- Hyperkalaemia (>24 h after burns or spinal injury)
- Severe muscle pains
- Prolonged paralysis

3.6 Passage of Tube

The aim is to be swift but not rushed. The whole process should take no more than 1 min.

The vocal cords are attached anteriorly to the thyroid cartilage and posteriorly to the arytenoid cartilages (Figs. 3.12 and 3.13). The view is described by the Cormack and Lehane classification (Fig. 3.14). A modification divides grade 2 into: grade 2a: part of the vocal cords are seen and 2b: only the arytenoids seen. This should be recorded along with additional equipment required (e.g., McCoy blade) and handed over to other medical personnel, indicating the difficulty or otherwise of intubation.

A poor view may be improved by Backward Upward (pushing an anterior larynx backwards and then up towards the laryngoscope) Rightward (as the laryngoscope is coming

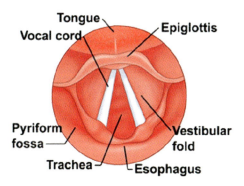

FIGURE 3.13. Laryngoscopy and laryngeal inlet Reproduced with kind permission from the Anaesthesia UK website.

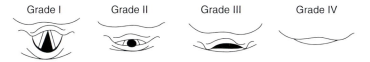

FIGURE 3.14. Cormack and Lehane intubation grade. Reproduced with kind permission Anaesthesia UK Website.

in from the right side of the mouth/tongue) Pressure (BURP) on the thyroid and cricoid cartilages together.

3.6.1 Laryngoscope

A Macintosh size 3 laryngoscope is suitable for most adults and is easier to insert than a size 4 when mouth opening is limited. A size 4 may be required in patients with a large jaw. Care should be taken not to insert a size 4 too far initially as it is easy to pass the larynx and reach the esophagus which can be difficult to recognize for the inexperienced. A McCoy blade, which has a flexible tip, (Fig. 3.15) has been shown to significantly improve the view at laryngoscopy when the neck is immobilized (Gabbott 1996). There is therefore an argument for using one routinely in the pre-hospital environment. Unfortunately they are not currently available in disposable form and require appropriate cleaning between patients. Other airway devices such as the "Airtraq" may also provide an improved view and reduce the time to successful intubation (Maharaj et al. 2007). Personnel should have experience of using these devices before attempting to use them for PRSI.

3.6.2 Bougie

A gum elastic bougie (or disposable tracheal introducer of a similar design) should be used electively in all cases due to the increased incidence of difficult intubation (Figs. 3.16– 3.19). If only the arytenoids are visible correct placement should be straightforward and even when only the epiglottis is seen this can be used as a landmark to guide the blind placement of a bougie. The "click" of the tip of the bougie passing over the tracheal cartilages may be felt confirming correct placement. Alternatively, resistance may be felt as the bougie reaches the carina or bronchi, whereas it will generally pass unhindered down the length of the esophagus. The latter technique can only be used if the bougie is used independently then the ETT railroaded over afterwards by the

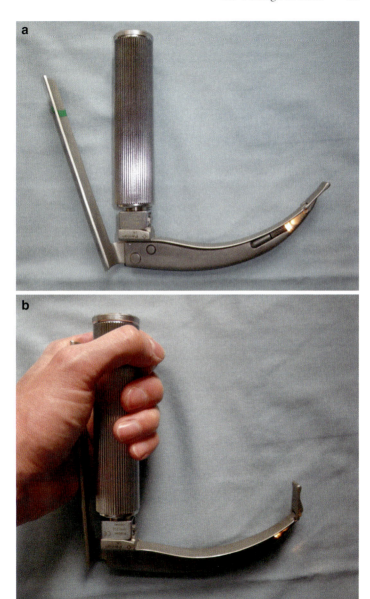

FIGURE 3.15. (a). Initial 'resting' position for insertion of blade into vallecula. (b). Tip flexed by closing lever to lift epiglottis.

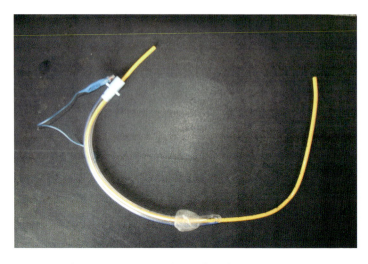

FIGURE 3.16. An ETT mounted on a bougie.

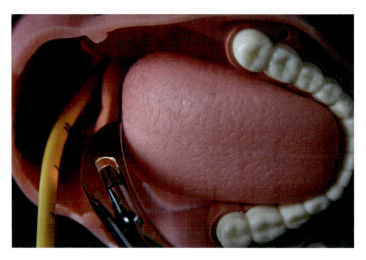

FIGURE 3.17. The use of a bougie as a guide for the passage of an ETT.

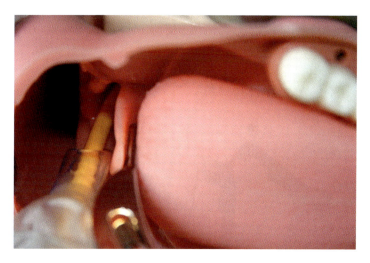

FIGURE 3.18. An ETT being passed over a bougie with the tip of the laryngoscope in situ.

assistant. The alternative technique of preinserting the bougie in the tube requires the bougie to be held firmly below the tip of the ETT to allow control of the tip. This is best understood by practice on a mannequin.

The ETT will sometimes be held up as the tip catches on the vocal cords. This can be resolved by rotating the ETT anticlockwise 90° in the majority of cases. Occasionally cricoid pressure will need to be released.

The incidence of complications markedly increases after two failed attempts at passing an endotracheal tube (Mort 2004). For this reason, after two attempts the failed intubation drill is followed. It is only worth attempting intubation for a second time if something is going to be changed for the second attempt e.g., different size blade, McCoy laryngoscope, position of the patient. Repeating exactly the same maneuver will only give the same view and delay the establishment of adequate oxygenation/ventilation by another means. Ventilation should be carried out between attempts if required to maintain SpO_2 above 92%.

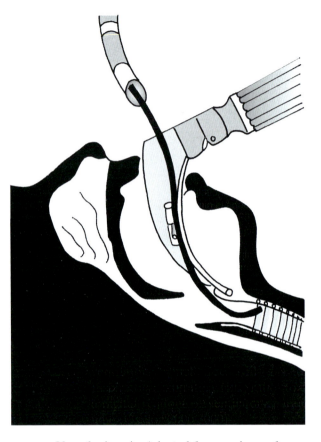

FIGURE 3.19. Use of a bougie. Adapted from an image from www.anesthesiologists.org, with kind permission.

3.6.3 Plan A and Plan B

When embarking on an RSI it is essential to be clear not only about your primary objective but also to have a prepared fallback position should things go wrong. In the prehospital environment, when faced with a failed intubation, "waking the patient up" is unlikely to be clinically appropriate (Box 3.8).

> # Box 3.8 Planning for PRSI
>
> - *Plan A* - A successful rapid sequence intubation
> - *Plan B* - A contingency for "failed intubation"

3.6.4 Failed Intubation Drill (Appendix "Failed Intubation Protocol")

In the event of a failure to intubate during PRSI a well-rehearsed drill should increase the likelihood of a good outcome. The intubator should rapidly recognize that the situation requires the implementation of the "Failed Intubation Drill" and should declare this to the assistant. The assistant should then immediately release cricoid pressure and pass the LMA (Appendix "Use of the Laryngeal Mask Airway") or other supraglottic device. If a LMA is used there are advantages to using one which allows higher ventilation pressures to be delivered e.g., Proseal™ LMA. The selection of secondary device depends upon the intubators familiarity of use. The assistant should then immediately prepare the surgical cricothyroidotomy kit in case this is required. If ventilation is unsuccessful with the rescue device, ventilation with a BVM and guedel airway should be attempted, whilst the most experienced team member performs a surgical cricothyroidotomy (Appendix "Emergency Cricothyroidotomy"). A second dose of suxamethonium should not be used, as it can induce a profound bradycardia.

3.7 Post Intubation

3.7.1 Confirmation of Placement

Unrecognized esophageal intubation is a preventable and catastrophic complication of PRSI. The gold standard for ensuring correct ETT positioning is the presence of $ETCO_2$ using capnography.

3.7.2 Capnography

Battery powered, lightweight and easily portable monitors are commercially available. They use infra-red absorbance spectroscopy to determine the presence and quantity of CO_2 in the exhaled breath. They either display this information as a figure (capnometer) or as a waveform (capnograph). The waveforms can be useful for the recognition of trends in ventilation and diagnosing ventilatory problems. These devices may need regular calibration and are less useful in diagnosing esophageal tube place after cardiac arrest when little if any carbon dioxide is being produced.

3.7.3 Colorimetric Capnometer

This is a lightweight device that attaches to the end of the endotracheal tube. It consists of a filter paper impregnated with a pH-sensitive, non-toxic chemical indicator that reversibly changes color on contact with CO_2. The Easy Cap™ is an example of this device. It provides a breath to breath color change from purple on inspiration to yellow on expiration confirming the presence of CO_2 in the exhaled breath. It is the simplest and most reliable (it requires no batteries) method of confirming placement in the trachea.

Other methods are used to confirm correct placement, but can be misleading and are not infallible. These include:

Visual Confirmation: The ETT may be seen to pass through the cords. Unfortunately the view is often not ideal and when railroading the tube, any view one had of the larynx, may be blocked by the passing tube.

Auscultation: Listening (in both axillae) with a stethoscope may confirm air entry in the lungs. It will also confirm bilateral ventilation and confirm that the tube has not been inserted too far i.e., into the right main bronchus. Unfortunately breath sounds can be difficult to hear in some patients (e.g., obese, emphysema) and this is often exacerbated in the pre-hospital environment due to external noise.

Look and Feel: Chest movement may be seen or felt with hands placed on the chest. This is not very reliable.

Esophageal Detector: There are commercial devices based on the "Wee sophageal detector." These are essentially large syringes that are attached to the ETT, and an attempt is made to rapidly withdraw air. If the tube is in the trachea, this is easy to do, if in the esophagus, resistance is felt due to collapse of the compliant walls of the esophagus. This technique can be reassuring in patients in cardiac arrest where no carbon dioxide is being produced and is therefore not detected convincingly by any of the methods described earlier. It is very accurate in adult patients, however false positives can occur in very obese patients and children due to collapse of the trachea.

References

Benumof JL, Dagg R, Benumof R (1997) Critical hemoglobin desaturation will occur before a return to an unparalyzed state following 1mg/kg intravenous succinylcholine. Anaesthesiology 87:979–982

Cook TM (1996) Cricoid pressure: are two hands better than one. Anaesthesia 51:365–368

Crosby ED (2006) Airway management in adults after cervical spine trauma. Anesthesiology 104:1293–1318

Fakhry SM et al (2006) Prehospital rapid sequence intubation for head trauma: conditions for a successful program. J Trauma 60:997–1001

Flucker CJ, Hart E, Weisz M, Griffiths R, Ruth M (2000) The 50 millilitre syringe as an inexpensive training aid in the application of cricoid pressure. Eur J Anaesthesiol 17:443–447

Gabbott DA (1996) Laryngoscopy using the McCoy laryngoscope after application of a cervical collar. Anaesthesia 51:812–814

Gataure PS, Vaughan RS, Latto IP (1996) Simulated difficult intubation. Comparison of the gum elastic bougie and the stylet. Anaesthesia 51:935–938

Goutcher CM, Lochead V (2005) Reduction in mouth opening with semi-rigid cervical collars. Br J Anaesth 95:344–348

Greaves I, Porter KM, Revell MP (2002) Fluid resuscitation in pre-hospital trauma care: a consensus view. J R Coll Surg Edinb 47:451 457

Greaves I, Porter KM, Ryan JM (eds) (2000). Shock. In: Trauma care manual. London, Arnold, pp 78–79

Haslam N, Parker L, Duggan JE (2005) Effect of cricoid pressure on the view at laryngoscopy. Anaesthesia 60:41–47

Hasting RH, Wood PR (1994) Head extension and laryngeal view during laryngoscopy with cervical spine immobilization maneuvers. Anaesthesiology 80:825–831

Heath KJ (1994) The effect of laryngoscopy on different cervical spine immobilization techniques. Anaesthesia 49:843–845

Herman NL, Carter B, Van Decar TK (1996) Cricoid pressure: teaching the recommended level. Anesth Analg 83:859–863

Maharaj CH, Buckley E, Harte BH, Laffey JG (2007) Endotracheal intubation in patients with cervical spine immobilization: a comparison of macintosh and airtraq laryngoscopes. Anesthesiology 107:53–59

May P, Trethewy C (2007) Practice makes perfect? Evaluation of cricoid pressure task training for use within the algorithm for rapid sequence induction in critical care. Emerg Med Australas 19:207–212

Mort TC (2004) Emergency tracheal intubation; complications associated with repeated laryngogoscopic attempts. Anesth Analg 99:607–613

Murray GD et al (2007) Multivariable prognostic analysis in traumatic brain injury: results from the IMPACT study. J Neurotrauma 24:329–337

Newton A, Ratchford A, Khan I (2008) Incidence of adverse events during prehospital rapid sequence intubation: a review of one year on the London Helicopter Emergency Medical Service. J Trauma 64:487–492

Noguchi T, Koga K, Shiga Y, Shigematsu A (2003) The gum elastic bougie eases tracheal intubation while applying cricoid pressure compared to a stylet. Can J Anaesth 50:712–717

Nolan JP, Wilson ME (1993) Orotracheal intubation in patients with potential cervical spine injuries. An indication for the gum elastic bougie. Anaesthesia 48:630–633

Owen H, Follows V, Reynolds KJ, Burgess G, Plummer J (2002) Learning to apply effective cricoid pressure using a part task trainer. Anaesthesia 57:1098–1101

Practical guidelines for management of the difficult airway (1993) A report by the American Society for Anasthesiologists Task Force on Management of the Difficult Airway. Anaesthesiology 78:597–602

Sellick BA (1961) Cricoid pressure to control regurgitation of stomach contents during induction of anaesthesia. Lancet 2:404–405

Smith C, Dejoy SJ (2001) New equipment and techniques for airway management in trauma. Curr Opin Anaesthesiol 14:197–209

Vanner RG, Asai T (1999) Safe use of cricoid pressure. Anaesthesia 54:1–3

Vanner RG, Clarke P, Moore WJ, Raftery S (1997) The effect of cricoid pressure and neck support on the view at laryngoscopy. Anaesthesia 52:896–900

Wang HE, Davis DP, Wayne MA, Delbridge T (2004) Prehospital Rapid-Sequence Intubation-what does the evidence show? Prehosp Emerg Care 8:366–377

Xeropotamos NS, Coats TJ, Wilson AW (1993) Prehospital surgical airway management: 1 year's experience from the Helicopter Emergency Medical Service. Injury 24:222–224

Chapter 4
Post-intubation Management

At the end of this chapter you should:

- Understand the importance of post-intubation care
- Know the ABCDE approach to pretransfer checks

The quality of care delivered after intubation and during transfer to hospital may have as much influence on outcome as the intubation itself. Experience from intrahospital transfers suggests that unexpected problems or complications occur during 62–68% of transfers (Lovell et al. 2001) (Papson et al. 2007). Critical or life-threatening incidents occurred in nearly 9%. In the prehospital environment the incidence of complications can be expected to be higher as the environment is often less controlled and the patient more unstable (intrahospital transfers usually only take place if patients are relatively stable). Lovel commented that many of the difficulties were preventable with adequate pretransport communication and planning.

Intubating a patient increases the burden of patient monitoring and complicates the transfer. The patient can no longer protect their own airway, they are unable to ventilate themselves effectively or communicate the potential for deterioration or further injury. Additional equipment is required to adequately monitor their vital signs and ventilation. Vigilance is essential to avoid accidental extubation, disconnection, and

A. Griffiths et al., *Pre-Hospital Anaesthesia Handbook*,
DOI: 10.1007/978-1-84996-159-2_4,
© Springer-Verlag London Limited 2010

decannulation. It is possible to minimize these risks by careful packaging and meticulous monitoring during the transfer to hospital. Minimum monitoring standards are essential for the safe transfer of intubated patients in the prehospital environment. This should ideally include both visual and audible alarms (through helmet/headsets on aircraft) for both ventilation and standard monitoring equipment.

Long distance transfer of critically ill patients can be achieved without any major complications in the setting of a dedicated transfer team (Uusaro et al. 2002). It is reasonable to assume that a dedicated and well-trained prehospital team should also minimize, if not eliminate, the incidence of major complications on route to hospital. The transfer of intubated patients between hospitals, is usually carried out by anesthetists (Jameson and Lawler 2000), but a large number of prehospital intubations and subsequent transfers are not. For non-anaesthetists who are not used to transferring critically ill ventilated patients there is a lot to remember, but an ABCDE approach should make this easier. This system is also valuable for those who consider themselves experienced transfer doctors. The stress of managing a critically ill patient in a prehospital environment can easily result in incomplete preparation and an increased risk of adverse events.

Pretransport planning and preparation in a structured manner is therefore the focus of this chapter. After intubation and before transfer a full check should be performed.

4.1 A (and c-Spine) BCDE Approach

4.1.1 Airway

The airway only remains protected as long as the endotracheal cuff remains inflated below the vocal cords. For this reason the endotracheal tube must be secure. This can be achieved using either adhesive tape or a fabric tie. Both techniques have their limitations. Tape is unlikely to provide adequate security in the presence of rain, sweat, grease, blood, or facial hair. Fabric tube ties overcome these issues, however, if applied too tightly, can lead to venous congestion and increased intracranial pressure. For this reason, tape should be used preferentially for head injured patients.

Flexion and extension of the head can lead to migration of the endotracheal tube. This is particularly relevant in children where smaller anatomy means that relatively small movements can result in either endobronchial intubation or extubation. Although in children, flexion appears to consistently cause downward displacement of the tube (distance relative to age) and extension causes upward movement, in adults the movement can be either way (up to 2 cm down or 3 cm out) (Weiss et al. 2006; Yap et al. 1994). In an adult the endotracheal tube cuff should be placed 2 cm below the cords to minimize the risk of problems occurring in either direction. Some endotracheal tubes are marked at the distal end to provide an indication of optimal positioning. The mark on the tube should usually be positioned just through the vocal cords.

The left main bronchus is narrower and branches off the trachea at more of an acute angle compared with the right; hence endobronchial intubation is invariably right sided. The incidence of endobronchial intubation can be reduced by ensuring the presence of bilateral breath sounds and chest movement after securing the tube in position. Endobronchial intubation should be suspected in the presence of unexpectedly high airway pressures during ventilation. Bronchospasm may also be an indicator of endobronchial intubation or the potential for it (the bronchospasm may be due to carinal irritation). Withdrawing the endotracheal tube by 2 cm is usually adequate to improve the situation.

When the ETT is positioned satisfactorily, note the measurement at the teeth (usually 22 cm for an adult male). This may then be used as a reference point if there are concerns that the tube has migrated during transfer. This information should be recorded and communicated on handover.

Prolonged endotracheal tube cuff inflation pressures of greater than 30 cm H_2O can lead to tracheal mucosa ischaemia (Seegobin and van Hasselt 1984). This is unlikely to be an issue during transport following PRSI within the UK due to relatively short transfer times. If longer journey times are expected (particularly by air, when cuff pressure is proportionately greater than capillary pressure will increase relative to capillary pressure), consideration should be given to monitoring and adjusting pressures with a simple hand-held device. Alternatively the air can be exchanged for saline, although it can be difficult to adjust cuff pressure using saline.

Effective suction must always accompany the intubated patient. Both Yankauer (oropharyngeal) and endobronchial catheters should be available for airway toileting en route.

A heat moisture exchange filter (HMEF) should always be used between the patient and the ventilator circuit. This protects the ventilator equipment from contamination and allows some moisture and heat exchange between the inspired and expired gases. Cold dry inspired gases can increase heat loss and degrade the function of respiratory cilia (Box 4.1).

Box 4.1 Post-intubation airway check

- Secure tube
- Check position
- Suction available
- HMEF

4.1.2 Cervical Spine

One in every nine trauma patients requiring intubation will have a cervical spine injury. Of these, one third will be unstable (Patterson 2004). It is the custom and practice of prehospital staff in the UK to use a semi-rigid collar and long spinal board for extrication and transfer of appropriate trauma casualties. Prolonged periods of immobilization on a spinal board can lead to the development of pressure necrosis. This is more likely to occur in the hypotensive patient. The skin overlying bony prominences in contact with the spinal board is most at risk (scapulae, sacrum, and heels). The long spinal board is also not a good spinal splint as it allows a significant degree of lateral movement. Therefore it should be considered only as an extrication device. If transfer times are likely to be prolonged (e.g., >30 min), the patient should be "scooped" onto a vacuum mattress and the spinal board used purely for supporting the mattress during transfer between vehicles/trolleys. When a patient is transferred on a long spinal board, it should be removed as soon as possible on arrival in the ED (i.e., on completion of the primary survey) (Vickery 2001). Semi rigid collars are also associated with significant morbidity. Inappropriate sizing can lead to raised intracranial pressure. It is important to ensure that no clothing is trapped under the collar as this may result in skin injury and inadequate stabilization. It is essential that correct sizing and fitting takes place on scene because these collars often remain in situ for a considerable time prior to definitive management and hospital staff may have limited experience in their use (Box 4.2). Secure head blocks (or fluid/sand bags secured with tape) are also required to ensure full cervical spine immobilization.

Box 4.2 Post-intubation cervical spine check

- Collar sized and fitted correctly
- Consider vacuum mattress

4.1.3 Breathing

Manual ventilation cannot provide reliable and consistent minute ventilation (Cardman and Friedman 1997). It is also labor intensive and limits concurrent activity. Mechanical ventilators address both these issues, although operators should be aware that the delivered minute volume may differ by ±20% from the ventilator settings (Gerais et al. 1987). Even when mechanical ventilation is employed, optimal oxygenation and ventilation cannot be assured (Helm et al. 2003). End-tidal CO_2 can be used to judge the adequacy of ventilation. The normal $PaCO_2$–$EtCO_2$ gradient is between 0.3 and 0.7 kPa (Bhavani-Shankar et al. 1992). Unfortunately $ETCO_2$ is only predictive of the trend in $PaCO_2$ in 77% of ventilated patients.

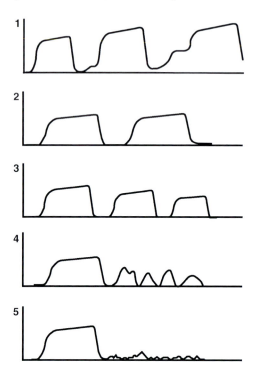

FIGURE 4.1. Typical Capnograph Traces. (1) Evidence of increasing cardiac output (and subsequent production of CO2/delivery to the lungs), (2) Typical steady trace, (3) Suggestive of falling cardiac output (4) Patient attempting to breathe (5) Disconnection.

A capnograph/capnometer is essential for monitoring end-tidal CO_2 during transfer. The waveforms can be useful for the recognition of trends in ventilation and diagnosing ventilatory problems.

4.1.4 Over Ventilation or Fall in Cardiac Output

Hypovolemic patients and patients with severe lung contusions are most likely to have a greater difference between

$PaCO_2$ and $ETCO_2$ (pathological increase in dead space). These patients may have gradients as high as 1.5 kPa. The delivery of carbon dioxide to the lungs is dependent primarily on pulmonary blood flow. If ventilator settings remain unchanged then an increase in $ETCO_2$ implies an improvement in total body cardiac output (Falk 1993). Similarly, a reduction in $ETCO_2$ should provoke a reassessment of the circulation before simply reducing the minute ventilation.

When using a mechanical ventilator a self-inflating bag-valve-mask must always be taken as a backup. It not only allows ventilation in the event of mechanical failure but can also be used to hand ventilate via the facemask in the event of accidental extubation. To ensure adequate oxygenation in this situation, it is necessary to have a flow meter adapter on one of the oxygen cylinders and oxygen tubing to fit the connector, attached to the bag. Modern lightweight cylinders will usually have both Schrader and "fir tree" connectors which makes things easier.

Before departure calculate the maximum oxygen requirement for the journey and confirm that sufficient is being carried (see under *ventilators* later). Make a note of the Peak airway pressure – if this changes during transfer, a problem is developing or has occurred (e.g., ETT moved into bronchus, tension pneumothorax, etc.).

Reassess the chest before starting the transfer. This is probably the last chance to auscultate the chest prior to arrival in hospital. The patient has been ventilated for a few minutes by this stage and if a tension pneumothorax is developing, it should be apparent by now. This allows appropriate management to take place prior to departure rather than during transfer (Box 4.3).

Box 4.3 Post-intubation breathing check

- Mechanical ventilator settings and oxygen requirements
- BVM available
- Reassess the chest

4.1.5 Circulation

Intravenous access should be checked for patency and security prior to transfer. A cannula falling out during transfer may be at best inconvenient and at worst a disaster. Reestablishing venous access whilst on the move is invariably difficult. A cannula should be secured with tape rather than just a dressing. Most dressings do not provide direct countertraction to the cannula being pulled out. They often simply lie over the top of the cannula, keeping the site clean. The cannula should be fixed so that it cannot be tugged out of the vein nor can it be lifted up from the skin and kinked over. In addition, the IV giving set tubing should be secured to the arm. Incorporating a loop provides additional protection.

The BP should be monitored closely during transfer, either by regular automatic cycling (3–5 min) or in ongoing hemorrhage, by palpation of the radial pulse.

Intubated trauma patients are a heterogeneous group. Age, physiological reserve, pattern, and severity of injury, and individual response to injury all differ. Similarly: entrapment, current physiological status, proximity to definitive care, and mode of transport all influence fluid administration decisions. As discussed earlier; the optimal prehospital fluid resuscitation strategy is not clear. Patients that are bleeding acutely can be separated into two groups: controllable and uncontrollable hemorrhage.

The controllable hemorrhage group includes soft tissue trunk injury and extremity trauma. In this group, hemorrhage can be controlled at scene by direct pressure, pressure dressings, proximal arterial pressure, and tourniquet. Fluid should be administered to these patients if evidence of hypoperfusion is present. The aim of management should be to achieve a good volume radial pulse and the improvement of $ETCO_2$ but not achieving normovolemia.

In the uncontrollable hemorrhage group, rapid transfer to definitive care is the key to survival. This should not be delayed by fluid administration or attempted further IV access. Fluid should be given if there is a marked reduction or loss of ETCO$_2$, loss of radial pulse, or bradycardia, as these signs suggest imminent cardiac arrest. Otherwise, fluids should be limited to keeping the vein open. A fluid bolus may also be considered if severe tachycardia or signs of heart strain are evident on the ECG.

The optimum choice of prehospital fluid is yet to be established. At present 0.9% saline given as a 250 mL bolus and titrated to response is recommended (Greaves et al. 2002). When weight and logistic considerations are important, 7.5% hypertonic saline (HS) may be considered. HS is thought to increase the intravascular volume by between 3 and 4 times the volume infused (small volume resuscitation). A bolus of 100 mL should be used and titrated to clinical effect. There are theoretical advantages to the use of hypertonic solutions. They are effective in reducing ICP and improving CPP when used for the treatment head injury but this effect has not been shown to improve outcome (Cooper et al. 2004). They may also modulate the stress response to injury. There is some evidence to suggest that early administration of HS in the care of polytrauma patients may increase survival (Signorini et al. 1999).

Burns casualties, crush injuries, and patients with blast injuries of the chest should be managed to achieve normal cardiovascular parameters, and will need significant amounts of fluid.

If fluids are appropriate, ensure that an additional bag is readily to hand if the current one is expected to run out during the transfer.

An ECG may be susceptible to interference during transfer; however it is part of minimum monitoring. If the pulse oximeter is not reading, the ECG will be providing the only visual representation of heart rate. ST segment changes may suggest hypoxia, reduced cardiac output, or an acute coronary syndrome. The ECG may also indicate that the cause of sudden hypotension is a dysrhythmia rather than hypovolemia. This may require treatment with cardioversion, rather than persisting blindly (and inappropriately) with fluid therapy.

It is also important to note that pelvic injuries are commonly underdiagnosed. These injuries can lead to catastrophic bleeding during transfer yet are very difficult to detect in the prehospital environment. "Springing" the pelvis is very insensitive and may cause marked hypotension if an unstable fracture is present, so cannot be advocated. In any trauma victim when pelvic injury cannot be excluded, a binder or pelvic sling should be applied as early as possible (Box 4.4).

Box 4.4 Post-intubation circulation check

- Secure IV access
- Monitor BP/pulse/ECG
- Fluids vs. no fluids

4.1.6 Disability

The safe transfer of an intubated patient requires adequate muscle relaxation for the duration of the transfer. This can be achieved using a long acting nondepolarizing muscle relaxant, e.g., vecuronium or pancuronium. Muscle relaxation will ensure absolute immobility and ventilator synchrony during transfer and this enhances patient stability. The main risk of paralysis for the patient is awareness. Being conscious, yet paralyzed and unable to communicate pain and discomfort (from either trauma or intubation) can be a very distressing experience. To prevent this, the use of paralysis also mandates the use of adequate sedation. Patients who have a low GCS prior to intubation should also be provided with some form of sedation for two reasons: firstly, improvements in oxygenation and cardiac output secondary to medical intervention may well result in improved cerebral oxygenation and subsequent improvement in the level of consciousness. Secondly, these patients will still mount a sympathetic response to the presence of an endotracheal tube in the trachea or to the manipulation of injuries during handling. These sympathetic responses may aggravate raised intracranial pressure or lead to myocardial ischemia.

Check and document pupil response prior to transfer (Box 4.5).

Box 4.5 Post-intubation disability check

- Paralysis AND sedation
- Protect eyes but monitor pupils

4.1.7 Exposure and Packaging

Performing a full secondary survey following PRSI is not appropriate. Any potential sources of bleeding (including long bone, abdominal, and pelvic injury) should have been identified. Ensure that no major injuries to the patient's back have been missed (particularly wounds which may indicate intrathoracic or intraabdominal injury). Generally speaking, hypothermia should now be avoided. The patient should be covered with blankets to both reflect heat and to deflect rain and wind. These must be secure, particularly if transfer is by helicopter when loose articles become a serious hazard.

During the transfer of a sedated and paralyzed patient it is the responsibility of the medical attendant to prevent further injury. This includes ensuring that the patient is securely strapped to the stretcher/spinal board prior to a move. Limbs are particularly at risk whilst carrying and fitting stretchers into ambulances and aircraft. They should also be sufficiently padded to prevent pressure necrosis or direct nerve injury (e.g., ulna nerve at the elbow), prior to longer transfers.

It is important to leave access to IV lines in case drugs need to be given urgently during transfer. Leaving the hand and wrist uncovered also permits easy assessment of the radial pulse if required.

Monitoring leads, fluid tubing, and blankets are all liable to be dragged across a patient's face and may cause corneal abrasion unless the eyes are protected (e.g., taped closed). It is important to remember in a head injured patient, that assessing pupillary size and response is an important part of ongoing care. Patients with head injuries should ideally be nursed with a 15° head-up tilt. This improves venous drainage and reduces ICP (Box 4.6).

Box 4.6 Post-intubation exposure check

- Assess for potential source of blood loss and injuries to the back
- Prevent exposure (allowing IV access)

Finally, before transferring the patient to hospital, a member of the team should phone the receiving hospital to warn them of your imminent arrival. This is particularly important when a full trauma team (including urgent radiology) are likely to be required as this allows time to call the necessary hospital staff to the Emergency Department.

4.1.8 Handover and Documentation

Despite the urgency of the situation; clear, comprehensive and contemporaneous records must be kept. The minimum information should include a MIST (and AMPLE history if available). Patient and next of kin information should also be handed over if known. An indication of the progress of the patient while in your care will give valuable information about the requirement for further investigation or intervention. Any critical events or difficulties, e.g., with intubation, should also be reported.

It is important to communicate effectively with the receiving team members and ensure that the tempo of resuscitation and management is not lost. A ventilated patient must only be handed over to an individual capable of caring for them, i.e., experienced anesthetist in most cases. If not available, the prehospital clinician should be prepared to remain with the patient for a period of time until a suitable doctor is available for handover.

After handover the team should clean their equipment and replenish their consumables so they are ready for further tasking. A duplicate full set of prepacked equipment may facilitate a rapid turn around (Box 4.7).

Box 4.7 MIST handover

- Mechanism
- Injury
- Signs and symptoms
- Treatment

References

Bhavani-Shankar K, Moseley H, Kumar AY, Delph Y (1992) End-tidal carbon dioxide. Can J Anaesth 39:617–632

Cardman E, Friedman D (1997) Further studies of manually operated self-inflating resuscitation bags. Anesth Anal 56:202–206

Cooper DJ, Myles P, McDermott FT, Murray LJ, Laidlaw J, Cooper G, Tremayne AB, Bernard SS, Ponsford J (2004) Pre-hospital hypertonic saline solution. JAMA 291:1350–1357

Falk JL (1993) End-tidal carbon dioxide monitoring during cardiopulmonary resuscitation. Advances in anaesthesia. Mosby-Yearbook, St. Louis, pp 275–288

Gerais HW, Eberele B, Konietzke D, Hennes HJ, Dick W (1987) Comparison of blood gases of ventilated patients during transport. Crit Care Med 15:761–763

Greaves I, Porter KM, Revell MP (2002) Fluid resuscitation in pre-hospital trauma care: a consensus view. J R Coll Surg Edinb 47:451–457

Helm M, Schuster R, Hauke J, Lampl L (2003) Tight control of pre-hospital ventilation by capnography in major trauma victims. Br J Anaesth 90:327–332

Jameson PPM, Lawler PG (2000) Transfer of critically ill patients in the Northern region. Anaesthesia 55:489

Lovell MA, Mudaliar MY, Klineberg PL (2001) Intrahospital transport of critically ill patients: complications and difficulties. Anaesth Intens Care 29:400–405

Papson JP, Russell KL, Taylor DM (2007) Unexpected events during the intra-hospital transport of critically ill patients. Acad Emerg Mcd 14:574–577

Patterson H (2004) Emergency department intubation of trauma patients with undiagnosed spinal injury. Emerg Med J 21:302–305

Seegobin RD, van Hasselt GL (1984) Endotracheal cuff pressure and tracheal mucosal blood flow: endoscopic study of effects of four large volume cuffs. Br Med J (Clin Res Ed) 288:965–968

Signorini D, Andrews P, Jones P et al (1999) Predicting survival using simple clinical variables: a study in traumatic brain injury. J Neurol Neurosurg Psychiatr 66:20–25

Uusaro A, Parviainen I, Takala J, Ruokonen E (2002) Safe long-distance interhospital ground transfer of critically ill patients with acute severe unstable respiratory and circulatory failure. Intens Care Med 28:1122–1125

Vickery D (2001) The use of the spinal board after the pre-hospital phase of trauma management. Emerg Med J 18:51–54

Weiss M et al (2006) Tracheal tube-tip displacement in children during head-neck movement-a radiological assessment. Br J Anaesth 96:486–491

Yap SJ, Morris RW, Pybus DA (1994) Alterations in endotracheal tube position during general anaesthesia. Anaesth Intens Care 22:586–588

Chapter 5
Equipment and Minimum Monitoring Standards

By the end of this chapter you should know:

- What constitutes minimum monitoring standards
- The equipment required to safely carry out a PRSI.
- How to set a ventilator
- How to perform an oxygen requirement calculation

5.1 Monitoring

The standard of care and monitoring during PRSI and subsequent patient transfer should be the same as is expected in the anesthetic room or in the intensive care unit. The Association of Anesthetists and the Intensive Care Society have published guidelines for the transfer of intubated patients (Association of Anaesthetists of Great Britain and Ireland 1996; Whiteleys et al. 2002) (Box 5.1).

Box 5.1 Minimum monitoring standards

- ECG
- Noninvasive blood pressure
- Pulse oximetry
- Capnography

A. Griffiths et al., *Pre-Hospital Anaesthesia Handbook*,
DOI: 10.1007/978-1-84996-159-2_5,
© Springer-Verlag London Limited 2010

In exceptional circumstances it may be necessary to downgrade monitoring for access or logistic reasons. Pulse oximetry and capnometry are considered an absolute minimum. It is permissible to transfer ventilated patients to and from vehicles with this reduced level of monitoring providing the patient has not been unstable.

5.2 Equipment

The prehospital medical team should have a range of equipment to cover all aspects of patient care. The following list includes only those items that are specifically required when performing PRSI (Box 5.2).

Box 5.2 Essential equipment for PRSI

- Laryngoscope handle and two laryngoscope blades (functioning light/batteries).
- Endotracheal tubes of appropriate size and length (lubricated) (Box 5.3).
- Suction apparatus with yankauer and flexible catheters + Magill's forceps.
- Gum elastic bougie (not stylet).
- 10 mL syringe for inflating the cuff.
- Stethoscope to check tube placement.
- Tape or tie to secure the endotracheal tube.
- Catheter mount.
- HMEF.
- Apparatus to ventilate the lungs (BVM and mechanical ventilator).

Equipment should also be immediately available for the management of difficult or failed intubation (Box 5.4).

Box 5.3 Suggested sizes and lengths
              for endotracheal tubes

Sizes: Male – 8.0–9.0   Female 7.0–8.0
              Children over 2 size = Age/4 + 4.5 cm
Length: Male 22–24 cm Female 20–22 cm
              Children over 2 years Age/2 + 12 cm
Notes: (1) Only open and cut tubes immediately prior to use
(do not cut tubes in airway burns, anaphylaxis or trauma).
(2) The cuff must always be tested prior to use.

Box 5.4 Equipment for difficult
              or failed intubation

• Laryngeal mask airway (e.g., Proseal™)
• Emergency cricothyroidotomy kit (see Appendix "Actions
  on Desaturation")
• McCoy Laryngoscope, Airtraq etc.

All items should be checked daily against a list and correct
functioning assured.

5.3 Ventilators

Transport ventilators range from the very simple to the complex and expensive versions that are essentially portable ICU
ventilators. The simplest ventilators are those that are gas
driven and require no electrical supply to function. These are
probably still the commonest found in use in the UK (e.g.,
Oxylog 1000, Parapac) (Fig. 5.1). Moving up from these are

7. Attach to patient and note the generated peak airway pressure

4. Set Max pressure Alarm

3. No Air Mix = 100% (Air Mix = 45-60% depending on ventilator)

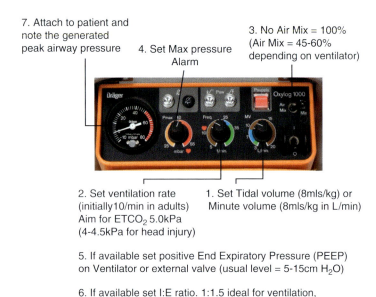

2. Set ventilation rate (initially10/min in adults) Aim for $ETCO_2$ 5.0kPa (4-4.5kPa for head injury)

1. Set Tidal volume (8mls/kg) or Minute volume (8mls/kg in L/min)

5. If available set positive End Expiratory Pressure (PEEP) on Ventilator or external valve (usual level = 5-15cm H_2O)

6. If available set I:E ratio. 1:1.5 ideal for ventilation, 1:2 or greater if hypovolaemic

FIGURE 5.1. Oxylog 2000 ventilator.

ventilators which are still gas driven but allow the Inspiratory:Expiratory (I:E) ratios to be adjusted and provide a digital readout of ventilatory parameters e.g., Minute volume (Oxylog 2000/3000) .

Gas driven portable ventilators consume oxygen at a rate in excess of the set minute ventilation. This varies between 0.5 and 1 L/min. It is essential for transferring personnel to be aware of the technical specifications (and battery life) of the ventilator in use and account for these during planning. This data is available from the user manuals.

The oxygen requirement for the duration of the transfer should be calculated prior to departure (Box 5.5) and sufficient cylinders carried (Box 5.6). If logistics permit, twice the calculated volume of gas should accompany the patient to allow for unexpected delay. If this is not possible, a one hour of reserve is the minimum acceptable.

Most ventilators possess a schraeder connector. Lightweight cylinders (e.g., CD size) have integral schraeder and fir tree connectors. Older cylinders must have a regulator attachment fitted. D and E size use a pin index regulator but the F size requires a bull nose connector. Different regulators and schraeder attachments must therefore be carried to ensure all cylinders are useable.

Box 5.5 How to perform an oxygen requirement calculation

Oxygen requirement = Ventilator dial setting (L/min) + Ventilator driving gas requirement (L/min) × Journey time (mins)

Ideally double the volume should be available

Box 5.6 Oxygen cylinder contents

D = 340 L (CD = 460 L)
E = 680 L
F = 1,360 L
Newer lightweight cylinders (e.g., CD, ZX) vary with make, therefore:

Always check the cylinder label!

5.3.1 How to set a ventilator (Fig. 5.1)

Ventilating patients with large tidal volumes (10–15 mL/kg) may lead to the release of inflammatory mediators (Slutsky and Tremblay 1998) and worsen Multiple Organ Dysfunction Syndrome (MODS) (Trembly et al. 1997). The adoption of a lung protective strategy in the intensive care unit appears to reduce mortality (The Acute Respiratory Distress Syndrome Network 2000). Critically ill patients intubated in the field are at risk of developing acute lung injury and MODS. For this reason, tidal volumes of 6–8 mL/kg body weight should be used. Peak airway pressures should be kept below 30 cmH$_2$O. If compliance is poor (airway pressures high relative to the tidal volume) the tidal volume should be reduced by 1 mL/kg to achieve this airway pressure. The ventilation rate should be set at between 6 and 30/min to achieve an ETCO$_2$ below 5.5 kPa. Usually a rate of 10–12/min is appropriate. For patients with head injury, the aim should be to achieve an ETCO$_2$ of 4–4.5 kPa.

Increasing minute volume will tend to reduce venous return, particularly in hypovolaemic patients. This may lead to a marked decrease in cardiac output. Animal studies suggest that achieving adequate oxygenation with the lowest possible minute volume will result in better cardiac output and blood pressure (Pepe et al. 2003); therefore, start with a rate of 6–8 in hypovolaemic patients. ETCO$_2$ in these patients should not be a concern.

In head injured patients with hypovolaemia a compromise may have to be made. Either: give additional fluid to maintain blood pressure whilst ventilating to a normal ETCO$_2$ and accept the risk of further bleeding, or, hypoventilate (e.g., six breaths per min) to allow improved hemodynamics and potentially better brain oxygenation (whilst closely monitoring pupil reaction for signs of increasing intracranial pressure subsequent to the increased PaCO$_2$) (Manley et al. 2000).

Positive end expiratory pressure (PEEP) can improve oxygenation in patients with chest pathology but may exacerbate the reduction in cardiac output and also increase ICP. PEEP is therefore not routinely used in patients with head injury during prehospital ventilation. However if SpO$_2$ is persistently low despite 100% oxygen the application of PEEP is appropriate and may have utility. Care should also be exercised in those with chest injury. The risk of tension pneumothorax increases with the onset of mechanical ventilation and PEEP. Marked deterioration during ventilation should be managed according to the desaturation protocol. If a tension pneumothorax is diagnosed it should be decompressed initially by needle thoracocentesis (Appendix "Needle Thoracocentesis"). Progression to a formal definitive decompression with either a tube (Schmidt et al. 1998) or open thoracostomy (Appendix "Thoracostomy") (Deakin et al. 1995) depends on the patient's response and the proximity to definitive care. Prophylactic chest drain insertion is not recommended.

The severe asthmatic patient can be very difficult to ventilate, and every effort should be made to get them to hospital without inducing anesthesia. If this is not possible do not apply PEEP, reduce ventilation rate and set I:E at 1:3 to allow time for expiration.

Hyperoxaemia (excessive oxygen in the blood) may be considered harmful in the critically ill population, but it is inappropriate to limit oxygen administration in the prehospital setting for this reason; avoidance of hypoxia is the priority. It may, however, be necessary to use lower concentrations of oxygen (e.g., "Air-mix") if supplies are limited. In this situation the aim is to keep SpO_2 above 93%. This equates to a PaO_2 of about 10 kPa in the majority of patients. The delivery of inspired oxygen concentration by portable ventilators may be completely variable or fixed (Air-mix/no-air mix setting). The air-mix setting can equate to a FiO_2 of 0.45 or 0.6 depending on the ventilator.

References

Deakin CD, Davies G, Wilson A (1995) Simple thoracostomy avoids chest drain insertion in pre-hospital trauma. J Trauma 39:373–374

Association of Anaesthetists of Great Britain and Ireland (1996) Recommendations for the transfer of patients with head injury to neurosurgical units. London

Manley GT et al (2000) Cerebral oxygenation during hemorrhagic shock: perils of hyperventilation and the therapeutic potential of hypoventilation. J Trauma 48:1025–1032

Pepe PE et al (2003) Emergency ventilatory management in hemorrhagic states: elemental or detrimental? J Trauma 54:1048–1057

Schmidt U, Salgo M, GericiiT, Blauch M, Maull KI, Tscherne H (1998) Chest tube decompression of blunt chest injuries by physicians in the field: effectiveness and complications. J Trauma 44:98–101

Slutsky AS, Tremblay LN (1998) Multiple system organ failure: is mechanical ventilation a contributing factor? Am J Respir Crit Care Med 157:1751–1755

The Acute Respiratory Distress Syndrome Network (2000) Ventilation with lower tidal volumes compared with traditional tidal volumes in acute lung injury and the acute respiratory distress syndrome. N Engl J Med 342:1301–1308

Trembly L, Valenza F, Ribeiro SP, Li J, Slutsky AS (1997) Injurious strategies increase cytokines and c-fos m-RNA expression in an isolated rat lung model. J Clin Invest 99:944–952

Whiteleys, Gray A, McHugh P, O'Riordan (2002) Transport of the critically ill adult. Intensive Care Society Standards, London

Chapter 6
Drugs and Sedation

By the end of this chapter you should be familiar with:

- The dilution, dosing and indications of the drugs routinely used for a PRSI
- The main side effects of these agents
- The aim of sedation and sedation end points

It is important that all members of the team are familiar with the dosing, dilution and side effects of the drugs used for PRSI regardless of their professional background. A small number of agents are chosen to develop familiarity and confidence in their use. All individuals involved with the drawing up and administration of these drugs must understand the pharmacology and interactions of these agents with the patient and other drugs.

6.1 Pre-Treatment

Some agents can be used to reduce the detrimental effects of laryngoscopy (hypertension, raised ICP). Fentanyl 1 mcg/kg can be used in physiologically robust patients with isolated head injuries and SBP > 120 mmHg. The peak effect is around 3 min after administration although respiratory depression may occur earlier than this, potentially giving a prolonged

A. Griffiths et al., *Pre-Hospital Anaesthesia Handbook*,
DOI: 10.1007/978-1-84996-159-2_6,
© Springer-Verlag London Limited 2010

period of hypoventilation prior to intubation. Alfentanil obtunds the response to laryngoscopy with a peak effect in 90 s and is relatively cardiostable (although may produce a bradycardia of vagal origin). The shorter onset time of Alfentanil potentially makes it a better option for RSI than Fentanyl. Ideally it should be administered 30 s prior to the induction agent. If respiratory effort is reduced the induction agent and muscle relaxant should be administered without delay.

There is currently no good evidence of benefit with the use of lignocaine to prevent exacerbation of intracranial pressure in head injury (Butler and Jackson 2002).

Children under 10 years may receive a prophylactic dose of 10 mcg/kg atropine to prevent suxamethonium induced bradycardia.

6.1.1 Fentanyl

This is a synthetic opioid. It is approximately 100 times more potent than morphine.

Indication	Attenuate response to laryngoscopy e.g., in isolated head injury
	Rapid acting (but relatively short-lived) analgesia
Presentation	Clear solution containing 50 mcg/mL (2 mL amp)
Dilution for use	Neat
Dose	1–2 mcg/kg IV
Onset	Peak effect 3 min
Offset	10–20 min
Side effects	Respiratory depression, Bradycardia, Hypotension
	Chest rigidity (high doses)

6.1.2 Alfentanil

This is a synthetic opioid. More rapid onset than fentanyl.

Indications	Attenuate response to laryngoscopy
Presentation	Clear solution containing 500 mcg/mL (2 mL amp)
Dilution for use	Neat
Dose	20 mcg/kg IV
Onset	Peak effect 90 s
Offset	5–10 min
Side effects	Same as fentanyl

6.1.3 Atropine

This is an anticholinergic.

Indications	Bradycardia due to increased vagal tone
	Cardiopulmonary resuscitation
	Organophosphate poisoning
Presentation	Clear solution 500 mcg/mL or 600 mcg/mL (1 mL amp)
	Or 3 mg in 10 mL autojet
Dilution for use	Made to 100 mcg/mL with saline
Dose	15–20 mcg/kg (3 mg required to block the vagus)
Onset	30 s
Offset	2–6 h

6.2 Induction Agents

Etomidate is advocated as the best induction agent for PRSI currently available (EMS Physicians 2006). Compared to other agents, it is relatively cardiostable. Propofol and thiopentone are the two most frequently used induction agents in hospital anesthesia, however, both can cause myocardial depression and significant hypotension.

Etomidate also reduces intracranial pressure and cerebral metabolism. With a minimal reduction in blood pressure, this means that cerebral perfusion pressure is maintained. This makes it an ideal choice for patients with head injury. Etomidate may induce temporary (12–24 h) adrenocorticol dysfunction. It has been shown to inhibit 11-beta hydroxylase production of cortisol, leading to mildly decreased serum cortical levels. This may be significant in sepsis (although steroid replacement easily resolves this), but does not appear significant in other patients.

Ketamine is another option for induction which is gaining popularity. Due to its sympathomimetic effect on beta-2 receptors it is particularly useful for induction of patients with severe bronchospasm. The beta-1 and alpha-1 effects can help to maintain blood pressure after induction however the induced tachycardia and hypertension can be a problem when trying to assess levels of sedation and hypovolemia. In elderly patients this may cause myocardial stress and ischemia. In younger hypovolemic patients it may be easier to use ketamine for sedation whilst maintaining a blood pressure, rather than combining midazolam with ephedrine.

Dissociative anesthesia occurs at higher doses (1–2 mg/kg). This is a state of dissociation from consciousness and the patient will appear in a trance or fugue state with their eyes open. At higher doses there is an increase in muscle tone and catalepsy (self-maintaining position). Airway reflexes and spontaneous respiration are usually preserved. Increased airway secretions and nausea can be a problem. Hallucinations on awakening from anesthesia can be an issue, and may be reduced by giving a small dose of midazolam.

6.2.1 Etomidate

This is a carboxylated imidazole.

Indication	IV induction of anesthesia
Presentation	Clear colorless solution for injection containing 2 mg/mL
Dilution for use	Neat in a 10 mL syringe
Dose	0.2–0.3 mg/kg
Onset	30 s
Offset	8–10 min
Side effects	Pain on injection (reduced by adding lignocaine)
	Myoclonus (abnormal movements) can be mistaken for seizure activity

6.2.2 Ketamine

This is a phencyclidine derivative.

Indications	Induction of anesthesia in patients with hypotension or asthma
	Potent analgesic; ideal for extrication
Presentation	Clear colorless solution containing 10, 50, or 100 mg/mL (caution)
Dilution for use	10 mg/mL (100 mg made up to 10 mL with saline)
Dose	Profound analgesia 0.25–0.5 mg/kg IV (1–4 mg/kg IM) IV induction 1–2 mg/kg IV (5–10 mg/kg IM)
Onset	30 s
Offset	5–10 min
Side effects	Emergence phenomenon hallucinations or unpleasant dreams during recovery. Incidence reduced by midazolam and recovery in a stimuli free environment.

Tachycardia and hypertension.
Contraindicated in ischemic heart disease.

May increase cerebral metabolism therefore relatively contraindicated in head injury.

Masseter spasm

Increased salivation

Increased upper airway reflexes. Instrumentation of the upper airway may lead to laryngospasm.

6.3 Muscle Relaxants

A muscle relaxant with rapid onset is required for PRSI. Suxamethonium is the most rapidly acting muscle relaxant currently available, and its effect wears off quickly. This may be an advantage in the 'can't intubate, cant ventilate' situation, as the patient may start to breath before critical hypoxia occurs. However, this 'wake up' option is rarely a luxury available to the pre hospital provider of anaesthesia, as the patient should not have been anaesthetised if it were possible to get them to hospital safely without intubation and ventilation. In this scenario it is far better to use an alternative airway technique.

To maintain paralysis a longer-acting relaxant is then required (Note: repeated doses of suxamethonium may cause severe bradycardia or asystole). Pancuronium is ideal as its duration of action (>1 h) mean that a second dose is rarely required. It also has a vagolytic effect which may counter the myocardial depressant effect of sedative drugs. It is, however, increasingly difficult to purchase. Atracurium is a shorter acting alternative, but requires refrigeration. Vecuronuim has a similar time profile to atracurium, does not need to be kept cool and has a lower incidence of anaphylaxis. It does however come as a powder which needs reconstituting before use. None of these drugs relax the muscles rapidly enough to be of use for the initial intubation. Rocuronium has been advocated for in hospital RSI. It has been shown to have a similar speed of onset to suxamethonium if used in high doses, but without many of the adverse effects. It does however take over 20 min to wear off, so the "wake-up" option is not present. Recently a novel reversal agent (sugamadex) for it has been marketed which may increase its popularity. This reversal agent is expensive.

The choice of muscle relaxants used will depend on the team and the system in which they are working. However it should be predetermined in system protocols, and regularly practised by the team members to ensure familiarity.

6.3.1 Suxamethonium

This is a depolarizing muscle relaxant.

Indications	Rapid onset paralysis as part of RSI
Presentation	Clear colorless solution containing 50 mg/mL (2 mL amp)
Dilution for use	Neat
Dose	1–1.5 mg/kg IV bolus
Onset	10–20 s
Offset	3–5 min usually
Side effects	Prolonged action (sux apnoea) in 4% lasts for 10 min to 2 h
	Fasciculations resulting in muscle pain
	Temporary raised intra ocular/cranial pressure
	Hyperkalaemia (burns and spinal cord injury) *but only >24 h after injury*
	Malignant hyperpyrexia (and masseter spasm)
	Bradycardia
	Anaphylaxis
Notes	Hydrolyses above 4°C so should ideally be stored in the fridge.

6.3.2 Pancuronium

This is a non-depolarizing muscle relaxant.

Indication	Maintenance of paralysis in an intubated patient
Presentation	Clear colorless solution containing 4 mg/mL
Dilution for use	Neat in a 2 mL syringe
Dose	Initial 0.1 mg/kg
	Supplementary dose 0.05 mg/kg
Onset	90–120 s
Offset	120 min
Side effects	Releases histamine

6.3.3 Atracurium

This is a non-depolarizing muscle relaxant.

Indication	Maintenance of paralysis in an intubated patient
Presentation	Clear colorless solution containing 10 mg/mL (5 mL amp)
Dilution for use	Neat in a 5 mL syringe
Dose	Initial 0.5 mg/kg
	Supplementary dose 0.1–0.2 mg/kg
Onset	90 s
Offset	20–30 min
Side effects	Releases histamine
Notes	Undergoes Hoffmann degradation and so should be stored at 2–8°C

6.3.4 Vecuronium

This is a non-depolarizing muscle relaxant.

Indication	Maintenance of paralysis in an intubated patient
Presentation	Lyophilized powder
Dilution for use	Diluted with 5 mL of water to yield a clear, colorless solution containing 2 mg/mL that is stable for 24 h
Dose	Initial 0.1 mg/kg
	Supplementary dose 0.05 mg/kg
Onset	2 min
Offset	14–30 min

6.3.5 Rocuronium

This is a non-depolarizing muscle relaxant.

Indication	Facilitate intubation and maintain paralysis in an intubated patient
Presentation	Clear colorless solution containing 10 mg/mL
Dilution for use	Neat in a 5 mL syringe
Dose	Intubation 0.6 mg/kg
	Supplementary dose 0.15 mg/kg
Onset	1 min
Offset	8–17 min
Side effects	Mild vagolytic

6.4 Sedation

Several agents can be used to sedate patients. Short acting agents e.g., propofol, must be given by infusion to avoid large variations in blood pressure. Bolus doses or large changes in infusion rate are not recommended as they can lead to cardiovascular instability. Infusion pumps, however, require batteries or an external power source and introduce an additional complexity to the handling of patients.

Longer-acting agents e.g., Midazolam can be administered by intermittent bolus dose. Bolus dosing of midazolam can also lead to hypotension; careful attention should be paid to the blood pressure after each bolus. It is recommended that a small dose should be given initially followed by careful titration depending upon patient response and blood pressure.

Ketamine may also be used for sedation by intermittent bolus, but effects on heart rate, blood pressure and cerebral metabolic rate mentioned earlier must be kept in mind (Box 6.1).

Box 6.1 The aims of sedation

- Prevent awareness/recall
- Prevent hypertension and tachycardia
- Reduce cerebral oxygen requirement

Adequate sedation may result in hypotension especially in hypovolemic patients. This effect is predictable and may be managed with a fluid bolus or bolus dose of a vasoactive drug e.g., ephedrine 3–6 mg. Care should be taken not to over treat, as surges of blood pressure may worsen hemorrhage (Box 6.2).

Box 6.2 Factors influencing the choice of sedative agent

- The familiarity of the individual with sedation technique
- Availability of an infusion pump (ideally required for shorter-acting drugs)
- The cardiovascular status of the patient (avoid propofol in hypotension and ketamine in hypertensive patients
- Chronic medical conditions
- The length of transfer (setting up an infusion for a short transfer may be inappropriate)
- The expected clinical course on arrival at definitive care

All individuals administering sedation should be familiar with the indications, dosing regime, contraindications and side effects of the agent used. Continuous vigilance is required for the signs inadequate sedation (Box 6.3).

Box 6.3 Signs of inadequate sedation

- Tachycardia
- Hypertension
- Dilated pupils
- Eye watering
- Sweating

A mix of morphine and midazolam has been recommended for sedation, 10 mg of each can be diluted in the same syringe to 10 ml.

Give 0.05–0.1 mg/kg (e.g., 3.5–7 ml), followed by repeated doses of 0.02 mg/kg (1–2 ml) during transfer, every 10–20 min as indicated. If an infusion device is available the intermittent bolus technique can be replaced by an infusion at an initial rate of 0.2 mg/kg/h.

6.4.1 Midazolam

This is a benzodiazepine.

Indications	Hypnosis and sedation
	Management of emergence phenomenon
	Anticonvulsant
Presentation	Clear colorless solution containing 5 mg/mL (2 mg/mL also available)
Dilution for use	2 mg/mL 10 mg diluted to 10 mL with saline
Dose	0.05–0.1 mg/kg (lower dose in elderly) initially 0.02 mg/kg maintenance bolus (1–2 mg in adults)
Onset	1–2 min but can take up to 15 min for maximal effect.
Offset	Variable and dose dependent but can be up to 2 h.
Side effects	Respiratory depression
	Hypotension
Notes	It can be used as an anticonvulsant. For these purposes bolus doses of 0.5–2 mg should be titrated to effect. It may be useful in the management of emergence phenomenon after ketamine administration but co-administration increases the likelihood of airway compromise.

6.4.2 Morphine

This is an opiate.

Indications	Analgesia
	Combined with midazolam for sedation
Presentation	Clear colorless solution 10 mg/mL (1 mL amp) (Beware 30 or 60 mg/mL 1 amp)
Dilution for use	1 mg/mL
Dose	0.05 mg/kg initially up to 0.2 mg/kg (titrated)
Onset	Peak effect after 15 min
Offset	2–4 h
Side effects	Respiratory depression, hypotension, urticaria, phlebitis

6.4.3 Propofol (2,6-Diisopropylphenol)

This is now the most commonly used induction agent in UK general anesthesia but is also widely used for sedation.

Indications	Induction and maintenance of general anesthesia
Presentation	White oil in water emulsion containing 10 mg/mL (1%) or 20 mg/mL (2%)
Dilution for use	Neat in a 50 mL syringe
Dose	1.5–2.5 mg/kg induction
	Intravenous maintenance of sedation at a dose of 1–4 mg/kg/h
Onset	15–20 s
Offset	5–10 min
Side effects	Pain on injection
	Induction may be associated with marked hypotension especially in patients with hypovolemia

6.5 Analgesia

6.5.1 Morphine

Morphine has long been the gold standard for the relief of severe pain in hospital and also for pre-hospital analgesia in the military. The benefits are that it provides good analgesia and the effect lasts for at least 2 h. The onset of morphine is relatively quick (a few minutes), however, the peak effect only occurs 15 min after administration. Therefore the potential exists to give repeated doses without waiting for the peak effect of the previous dose. This may result in respiratory depression which could manifest itself during transfer. Opiates are well suited for the provision of static analgesia. i.e., at rest with no external stimulation but are a poor choice for procedural analgesia.

6.5.2 Fentanyl

Fentanyl is an alternative to morphine. The onset and peak effect (3 min) is much quicker and this makes it an attractive choice. The offset is 20 min, which will provide adequate analgesia for short transfers; however, hospital staff may need to give further analgesia soon after arrival. For longer journeys it is advisable to administer morphine instead or in addition to the initial dose of fentanyl.

6.5.3 Entonox

Entonox is excellent for relief of short periods of extreme pain and is used widely in hospital medicine (e.g., during labor, relocating dislocated joints). The fact that it requires a compliant casualty and is contraindicated in suspected chest injuries limits its use in major trauma pre-hospital.

Entonox is a 50:50 mix of nitrous oxide and oxygen. It is administered via a demand valve, so requires adequate respiratory strength and patient compliance. It has a 30 s onset (so the casualty needs to breath the entonox for 30 s before the painful stimulus) and an offset of only 60 s. Other analgesia is usually required as well, with entonox used for any short periods of increased pain.

It has minimal cardiovascular, respiratory or neurological effects but is contraindicated when there would be a risk from expanding any gas filled space within the body (i.e., a pneumothorax). This is due to the fact that nitrous oxide will diffuse into the space faster than the nitrogen within the space can diffuse out leading to a buildup of pressure.

6.5.4 Ketamine

Ketamine is useful for managing relatively short periods of extreme pain when the nitrous oxide is contraindicated. It can provide adequate analgesia without loss of consciousness with a dose as small as 20 mg (0.25 mg/kg). Respiratory effort and blood pressure should be maintained during a period when the management of either may be difficult. For these situations it therefore has particular advantages over fentanyl or morphine. Ketamine is the drug of choice to provide dynamic analgesia i.e., analgesia suitable to facilitate intermittent intensely painful procedures.

6.5.5 Local Anesthesia (Appendix "Local Anesthetic Blocks")

Local anesthesia can occasionally be useful in the pre-hospital environment. A femoral nerve block can provide excellent analgesia for a femoral shaft fracture. It should ideally be used before applying a traction splint. Digital nerve blocks are simple to perform for dislocated fingers. Intercostal nerve blocks are rarely performed.

The volumes described in Appendix "Local Anesthetic Blocks" are for adult patients. Children require smaller volumes. Safe doses of local anesthetics for adults and children are:

| Lignocaine | 3 mg/kg | 1% lignocaine = 10 mg/mL |
| Bupivicaine | 2 mg/kg | 0.5% bupivicaine = 5 mg/mL |

6.6 Cardiovascular Support

6.6.1 Adrenaline

This is a catecholamine and acts as an inotrope, chronotrope and vasopressor.

Indications	Anaphylaxis
	Cardiac arrest
	Low cardiac output states
Presentation	Clear solution containing:
	0.1 mg/mL (1:10,000) 10 mL autojet or 1 mg/mL (1:1,000) 1 mL amp
Dilution for use (and dose)	*1:1,000* – 0.5 mL IM in anaphylaxis (0.1 mL/kg in children)
	1:10,000 – 10 mL in cardiac arrest (0.1 mL/kg in children)
	1:100,000 – 1 mL of 1:10,000 diluted to 10 mL with saline
	Use 1–2 mL boluses titrated to response in hypotension
Side effects	Dysrhythmia
	Tachycardia and myocardial ischaemia
	Lactic acidosis

6.6.2 Ephedrine

This is a sympathomimetic amine.

Indication	Hypotension
Presentation	Clear colorless solution containing 30 mg/mL (1 mL amp)
	Or 3 mg/mL (10 mL autojet)
Dilution for use	3 mg/mL (One ampoule 30 mg/mL up to 10 mL with saline)
Dose	3–6 mg (1–2 mL) titrated to response
Side effects	Dysrhythmia
	Tachycardia and myocardial ischaemia
	Vasoconstriction

References

Butler J, Jackson R (2002) Lignocaine premedication before rapid sequence induction in head injuries. Emerg Med J 19:554
National Association of EMS Physicians (2006). Prehosp Emerg Care 10:260

Further Reading

Sasada M, Smith S (1997) Drugs in anaesthesia and intensive care, 2nd edn. Oxford Medical Publications, Oxford

Chapter 7
Special Circumstances

By the end of this chapter you should know the specific management issues associated with:

- Hypothermia
- Pediatrics
- Obstetrics
- Head injury
- Transferring patients by air

7.1 Hypothermia

This is defined as a core temperature less than 35°C. It is associated with a number of undesirable effects:

- Cardiovascular arrhythmias occur at 30°C, VF at 28°C
- Vasoconstriction making IV access difficult and increasing myocardial work
- Increase blood viscosity reducing tissue perfusion
- Thrombocytopenia – platelets sequestered in the liver and spleen
- Shift of oxygen hemoglobin dissociation curve to the left – worsening tissue oxygen delivery
- Reduced level of consciousness (unconscious at 30°C)

There is some evidence that mild therapeutic hypothermia (34°C) improves outcome after traumatic brain injury in certain patients (Peterson et al. 2008). Hypothermia maintained

A. Griffiths et al., *Pre-Hospital Anaesthesia Handbook*,
DOI: 10.1007/978-1-84996-159-2_7,
© Springer-Verlag London Limited 2010

after out of hospital VF cardiac arrest is now accepted therapy to improve neurological outcome (European Resuscitation Council 2005). However patients with multiple trauma and no head injury have been shown to have a markedly worse outcome if they are allowed to become cold. In this patient group a core temperature of <32°C is invariably fatal (Jurkovich et al. 1987).

Coagulation depends on enzymes which function best at 37°C. Hypothermia therefore impairs blood clotting and will potentially result in increased blood loss in trauma patients.

It is not usually possible to increase core temperature in the pre-hospital environment. Management should be aimed at minimizing further heat loss.

In summary:

1. Cardiac arrest with return of circulation but remaining unconscious and no active bleeding – encourage cooling (unless hypothermic <34°C already).
2. Head injury with *no other significant trauma* – if GCS <8 encourage cooling.
3. All other patients – maintain temperature with blankets, etc.

7.2 Pediatrics

There is as yet no evidence to support the assumption that PRSI is superior to BVM for the treatment of children less than 12 years or weighing less than 40 kg in terms of survival or neurological outcome after injury. The only randomized controlled trial is poor quality, looks at non-drug assisted intubation and is inconclusive (Gausche et al. 2000). However as most pre-hospital doctors will have limited, if any experience, of anesthetizing children, and as children desaturate much more quickly than adults when they stop breathing, the threshold for PRSI is generally higher than for adults.

If the age of the child is known at dispatch then drug doses can be calculated en-route to the scene (drug dose calculators and Broselow tapes are available).

TABLE 7.1 Comparing infant and adult airways.

	Infant	Adult
Tongue	Relatively larger	Relatively smaller
Larynx	Opposite second and third cervical vertebrae	Opposite fourth, fifth, and sixth cervical vertebrae
Epiglottis	"U" shaped, large, floppy	Flat, flexible, erect
Hyoid/thyroid separation	Very close	Further apart
Smallest diameter	Cricoid ring	Vocal cord aperture
Consistency of cartilage	Soft	Firm
Shape of head	Pronounced occiput	Flatter occiput

A child is not a miniature adult and a more considered approach should therefore be taken when preparing for intubation. The pediatric airway differs significantly from the adult airway (Table 7.1). This requires an alteration in intubation technique.

The airway is smaller and as a result requires increased dexterity for manipulation and specialized equipment. The tissues of the airway are softer and more pliable. This means airway obstruction is more likely at extremes of head position and with apparent insignificant external pressure, especially under the chin when supporting a face-mask. The pronounced occiput may require support underneath the shoulders to achieve the sniffing position. (Children under 9 years old may suffer excess neck flexion in the neutral position.) The relative increase in the size of the tongue may make it more difficult to sweep and displace during the laryngoscopy. Using a curved blade in the vallecula may still leave the "floppy" epiglottis hanging down over the vocal cords obstructing the view. Going behind the epiglottis and lifting it with the tip of the blade is appropriate in these cases. The arytenoids in infants slant away from the intubator during laryngoscopy. This may prevent the endotracheal tube from passing easily. A 90° anti-clockwise rotation usually remedies this. If this is not the case, a smaller size tube maybe required.

The cricoid ring is the narrowest part of the pediatric airway. An endotracheal tube that is too large may pass through the cords, but not the cricoid ring. In these cases a smaller tube should be selected. All manipulations of a pediatric airway must be much gentler than in an adult as the structures are delicate and prone to edema. An infant's airway is typically 3 mm in diameter. A 1 mm circumferential swelling leaves an airway 1 mm in diameter. This is a 68% reduction. The same degree of oedema in an adult airway will only reduce the diameter by 25%.

Uncuffed endotracheal tubes have traditionally been used in children less than 10 years of age. This allows the use of a larger diameter tube minimizing airway resistance and maximizing airway toilet. It is important to ensure that a leak is present above 15 cm H_2O to prevent excessive pressure on the mucosa. Aspiration is less likely as the cricoid ring has a round aperture that should seal around the endotracheal tube. More recently, cuffed endotracheal tubes have been advocated. They may be beneficial with chest injuries when relatively high ventilation pressures are required.

Endobronchial intubation is very common in pediatric intubation. It should be expected and excluded by auscultation. Once a satisfactory position is confirmed, the length at the lips should be noted and the tube firmly secured. Head/neck movement should be avoided as this can cause the tube to move significantly both up and down the trachea, potentially leading to partial extubation or endobronchial intubation.

It is not uncommon for children to have loose teeth especially after trauma. Special attention should be paid to avoid aspiration of teeth during ventilation/intubation.

7.3 Obstetrics

The management of the pregnant trauma patient is emotionally charged as there are two lives potentially at risk. The preservation of the fetus is completely dependent on the effective assessment and resuscitation of the mother. Optimal management of the pregnant casualty requires an understanding of the physiological and anatomical changes that take place during pregnancy and how they impact upon PRSI.

From the first trimester there are marked changes in anatomy and physiology, due the increasing levels of progesterone from the placenta. They are widespread and include:

7.3.1 Airway

Increasing deposition of adipose tissue around the neck and breasts complicated by tissue edema, may make laryngoscopy and intubation more difficult. The risk of failed intubation for obstetric anesthesia is 1 in 300 (compared to 1 in 2,000 general surgical patients).

Gastric emptying and acidity are not changed by pregnancy. But the difference in pressure between the stomach and lower oesaphageal sphincter is reduced. During pregnancy, particularly with the onset of labor, administration of opiates or trauma may lead to an increased risk of reflux and loss of lower oesaphageal competence making aspiration more likely.

7.3.2 Breathing

The diaphragm may be displaced cephalad by up to 4 cm at term. This means that greater care should be exercised when performing thoracostomy in order not to cause diaphragmatic injury.

There is a 60% increase in oxygen demand during pregnancy, and a reduction in functional residual capacity of 20% which means that the onset of desaturation, even following pre-oxygenation, is rapid.

A rise in tidal volume of 40% results in a physiological hyperventilation and $PaCO_2$ of 4.0 kPa at term. An end-tidal CO_2 of 3.5–4.0 should be the goal to reflect physiological hyperventilation of pregnancy.

7.3.3 Circulation

Aorto-caval compression may occur when this pregnant uterus rests on the aorta or inferior vena cava. This reduces venous return and cardiac output as a result. Utero-placental blood flow is not auto-regulated and so is dependent on uterine blood flow. Even in the absence of maternal hypotension, uterine blood flow may be reduced by the supine position. After the twentieth week of gestation, uterine displacement should always be employed. In hospital this is usually achieved by tilting the operating table 15–30° to the left or placing a wedge under the right buttock. In the trauma patient, the most practical method is usually manual displacement of the uterus (literally pulling the abdomen over to the patient's left side, away from the inferior vena cava). A relative reduction in cardiac output may make the pregnant patient fell nauseous and vomit, even if the blood pressure is normal - this may also be accompanied by auditory/visual disturbances.

Cardiac output increases by 1–1.5 L/min and blood volume increases by up to 50% out of proportion with the increase in hemoglobin levels leading to a physiological anemia. The systolic and diastolic blood pressure falls by 5–15 mmHg during the second trimester and rises to normal levels at term. In the third trimester the resting heart rate increases by 15–20 beats/min. These physiological changes mimic the response to hypovolemia and may be misleading after trauma. In the presence of hypovolemic shock, shunting from the uterine and placental beds may occur. A blood loss of up to 1.5 L is therefore possible without any change in maternal physical signs. A fluid challenge should be considered in all pregnant trauma victims, as fetal hypoperfusion may be present despite normal maternal parameters.

Peripheral vasodilation makes veins more prominent. But in the presence of hypovolemia increased adipose deposition and edema can complicate IV access.

Pregnant women become hypercoagulable in the first trimester. Plasma concentrations of I, V, VIII, IX, X, and XII are all increased. Antithrombin III levels are depressed. This is the reason for the increased risk of pulmonary embolus in the first trimester.

7.3.4 Disability

If the level of consciousness is altered with no obvious cause, eclampsia (convulsions in pregnancy or following delivery in the absence of other causes) should be considered. Eclampsia almost always occurs in the presence of pre-eclampsia (hypertension, proteinuria and edema; with epigastric pain and low platelets in severe cases). In these cases fentanyl should be used to attenuate the sympathetic response to intubation.

7.3.5 Obstetric Referral

It is important to involve an obstetrician as soon as possible when dealing with pregnant trauma patients. Call ahead and alert the receiving hospital before departure. Useful information that should be conveyed includes:

1. Weeks of gestation (fundal height greater than 2 cm above the umbilicus suggests gestation greater than 25 weeks – and may be viable if delivered).
2. Mechanism of injury.
3. Obvious site of injury.
4. Vital signs on arrival and trends over time.
5. Interventions undertaken. If a PRSI has been undertaken the drugs given (esp. opiate dose and time) should be communicated as well as the cardiovascular stability during and after intubation.

7.4 Head Injury

Traumatic brain injury presents a particular challenge in the pre-hospital environment. Injury sustained on impact and prior to the arrival of the medical services is largely irreversible. The aim of management is therefore to avoid secondary injury (Box 7.1).

Box 7.1 Preventing secondary brain injury (Jones et al. 1994)

- The avoidance of hypoxia (PaO_2 >8 kPa or SpO_2 >92%).
- The avoidance of hypotension (keep SBP>90 mmHg or good volume radial pulse).
- The avoidance of hypercapnia ($ETCO_2$ of between 4 and 4.5 kPa).
- The avoidance of hyperglycemia (2.5> BM <10).
- The maintenance of plasma osmolality.

Hypercapnia causes a predictable increase in cerebral blood flow that leads to increased intracranial pressure. This may have a deleterious effect on outcome in head injured patients with poor intracranial compliance. Conversely, excessive hyperventilation should be avoided because hypocapnia causes cerebral vasoconstriction, which may lead to ischemia in areas of the brain that have the potential to recover. To avoid this, $ETCO_2$ should be kept between 4 and 4.5 kPa (aiming for a low/normal $PaCO_2$ of 4.5–5.0 kPa). Patients with physical findings suggestive of dangerously high ICP e.g., bradycardias, dilated pupil(s), may be temporarily hyperventilated to prevent coning. The aim for deliberate hyperventilation should be an $ETCO_2$ of 3–3.5 kPa in a stable patient and 2–2.5 kPa in patients with hypovolemia or chest injury (Helm et al. 2003).

Poor outcome from brain injury is associated with blood glucose levels >10 mmol/L and neurological damage per se can result from blood glucose levels <1.5 mmol/L. It is possible to manage hypoglycemia in the pre-hospital environment but it is not recommended to attempt to treat hyperglycemia. Hyperglycemia should be treated early on arrival to definitive care.

As noted previously the head injured patient may benefit from mild hypothermia and also from hypertonic saline. Mannitol can be used (0.5 g/kg) if raised intracranial pressure is suspected, or if the pupils dilate. It is however difficult to store in cool climates as it will crystallize out of solution (if this happens, rewarming it should make it go back in solution – it can be put on the bonnet of a car with its engine running).

7.5 Transferring Ventilated Patients by Air

Aeromedical transport of the critically ill patient is a speciality in its own right, however many providers of pre hospital anaesthesia (in the UK) work out of helicopters. It is therefore important to have a basic understanding on how this mode of transport can effect the patient's physiology.

7.5.1 Altitude

Most prehospital evacuation is carried out at altitudes below 2,000 m, making the issues of gas expansion and cabin pressure relatively unimportant.

7.5.2 Temperature

It is usually possible to control the temperature of the cabin, although this can be more difficult in certain helicopters. This will only prevent heat loss, it will not raise the temperature of a hypothermic patient. It is essential that care is taken to avoid heat loss and aid heat retention as early as possible during patient contact. This is best achieved by removing wet clothing and covering the patient from head to toe in dry blankets as the situation allows.

7.5.3 Acceleration/Deceleration

A patient being transferred in a helicopter may experience linear and radial forces. Both these forces may affect cardiovascular stability. Linear forces occur along the long axis of the airframe and a casualty will experience fluid shifts along this axis that may result in hypotension and tachycardia. Radial forces occur due to change in direction and occur outward from the center of the turn. Linear forces are particularly significant during take-off and landing in a fixed wing aircraft. If the patient is positioned with head to the front, take-off may result in a significant period of reduced venous return in a relatively hypovolemic patient. A dramatic reduction in cardiac output and blood pressure may occur to the point of PEA. This effect can be reduced by fluid loading prior to take-off. If the patient is positioned feet forward, there will be a period of increased intracranial pressure during take-off that may be detrimental in a patient with traumatic brain injury. On landing the effect is not as pronounced or for as long.

7.5.4 Vibration

This is a characteristic feature of helicopter flight. It can lead to blurred vision, shortness of breath, motion sickness and fatigue. It can also interfere with the body's ability to auto-regulate. This is important in heat related casualties.

Vibration may lead to wound disruption, fracture movement and bleeding that may lead to increased requirements for analgesia, sedation and resuscitation.

Monitoring vital signs (clinically and by machine) can be impeded by vibration. Taking a pulse can become very difficult and monitors may suffer interference leading to unreliable data. The C-locking function which synchronizes the pulse oximeter with the ECG can be useful to get a better SpO_2 trace during transfer. Newer transport monitors have better software and tend to function better in this environment.

7.5.5 *Noise*

Listening to a chest is usually impossible in a helicopter due to the noise so a clinical assessment relies on visual inspection and palpation with reference to airway pressures on the monitor. It is important to listen to the chest following PRSI and before boarding a helicopter, as it is easier (and better) to pick up a developing pneumothorax and deal with it whilst on the ground.

Noise can cause damage to hearing even in unconscious patients and so ear protection should be provided. A spare headset may be available for conscious patients allowing communication during transfer. If not, it is important to explain to the patient that communication will be difficult, prior to leaving. Hand signals may be required to alert the medical team if the patient develops problems en route.

Communication between medical staff and also with the pilot is important, so all should have linked headsets.

References

European Resuscitation Council (2005) European resuscitation council guidelines for resuscitation 2005. Resuscitation 67:S1–S189

Gausche M, Lewis RJ, Stratton SJ et al (2000) A Prospective randomised study of the effect of out of hospital paediatric endotracheal intubation on survival on neurological outcome. JAMA 283:783–790

Helm M, Schuster R, Hauke J, Lampl L (2003) Tight control of pre-hospital ventilation by capnography in major trauma victims. BJA 90:327–332

Jones PA, Andrews PJD, Midgeley S et al (1994) Measuring the burden of secondary insults in head injured patients during intensive care. J Neurosurg Anesthesiol 6:4–14

Jurkovich GJ, Greiser WB, Luterman A, Curreri PW (1987) Hypothermia in trauma victims. An ominous predictor of survival. J Trauma 27:1019–1024

Peterson K, Carson S, Carney N (2008) Hypothermia treatment for traumatic brain injury: a systematic review and meta-analysis. J Neurotrauma 25:62–71

Chapter 8
Complications and Adverse Events

By the end of this chapter you should:

- Be familiar with the types and incidence of common complications associated with PRSI.
- Be able to diagnose and manage the common adverse events during transfer.

8.1 Complications

All interventions are associated with complications. Understanding the cause of these complications allows the operator to take steps to avoid them and this makes the procedure safer. The incidence of complications during pre hospital anaesthesia is difficult to establish, with quoted overall rates varying between 5 to 39%. It is possible that the absence of benefit from pre-hospital intubation may result from the complications during and after its performance. One study has suggested an increased mortality from head injury associated with pre-hospital hypotension and hyperventilation (Davis et al. 2004).

8.1.1 Immediate Complications (Box 8.1)

These result from the mechanical technique of laryngoscopy and intubation. Upper airway trauma to the teeth, pharynx,

A. Griffiths et al., *Pre-Hospital Anaesthesia Handbook*, 113
DOI: 10.1007/978-1-84996-159-2_8,
© Springer-Verlag London Limited 2010

Box 8.1 Cause and incidence of immediate complications

Complication	Incidence (%)
Upper airway trauma to the teeth, pharynx, larynx, trachea (Adnet et al. 1998	1–5
Esophageal intubation (Adnet et al. 1998)	6.4
Endobronchial intubation	
Adults (Adnet et al. 1998)	2.8
Pediatrics (Easley et al. 2000)	15
Exacerbation of spinal cord injury	<1
Increased risk of aspiration (Adnet et al. 1998)	5.6–34
Anaphylactic shock (Adnet et al. 1998)	0.3
Bronchospasm (Adnet et al. 1998)	0.8
CVS instability	
Arrhythmias and bradycardia (Thomas 2004)	1.6–21
Hypotension (Reid et al. 2004)	17
Cardiac arrest (Adnet et al. 1998)	4
Hypoxia (SpO_2 <92%)	
Overall (Thomas 2004)	22–70
MILNS	40

larynx, and trachea results from excessive force or improper use of the laryngoscope blade. This is often compounded when the intubation is difficult or hurried. Prolonged attempts at intubation expose patients to harmful physiological responses and increase risk of laryngospasm, bronchospasm and aspiration of oropharyngeal contents. An attempt to intubate should not exceed 45 s and may require intermittent airway suctioning.

8.1.2 Early Complications (Box 8.2)

These usually arise during transfer. The complications include endotracheal tube migration leading to accidental extubation or endobronchial or oesaphageal intubation. Twisting of the

Box 8.2 Early complications

Complication	Incidence (%)
Barotrauma (pneumothorax, surgical emphysema and pneumomediastinum) (Schwartz et al. 1995)	1
Incorrect endotracheal tube sizing	24
Cricothyroidotomy	1.1
Hypercapnia (Helm et al. 2002)	16
Hypocapnia (Helm et al. 2002)	41
Failed RSI (Norwood et al. 1994)	1.1–4
Death within 30 min (Schwartz et al. 1995)	3

ETT or excessive cuff inflation pressures may lead to mucosal damage and an increased risk of subsequent tracheal stenosis. It is important to use a sterile endotracheal tube and ensure that it is kept as clean as possible during intubation as it may well remain in situ for a significant period of time and can be an early source of chest infection.

8.1.3 Late Complications

These complications can arise as result of the severity of a patient's injury or as a result of immediate or early complications (Box 8.3).

Box 8.3 Late complications

Complications	Incidence (%)
Late deaths (Sivilotti and Ducharme 1998) (hypoxic tissue injury and MODS)	26
Aspiration pneumonia mortality (Kluger and Short 1999)	4

8.2 Adverse Events

There are two main adverse events that occur during transfer of a critically ill ventilated patient:

1. Hypoxia (low SpO_2)
2. Hypotension

It is important that to be able to rapidly recognize and manage the underlying problem causing either of these two events.

8.2.1 Hypoxia (Low SpO_2)

It is important to have an action plan to manage sudden patient desaturation (Appendix "Actions on Desaturation").

First check whether the saturation probe is on a finger and has a normal trace. It is not uncommon for the probe to be hanging off the finger or on the floor/tucked in the blankets. Reposition probe whilst continuing assessment. If the probe is on and working, move straight on to find the problem.

The problem area can be narrowed down by a simple question: "**Is the chest moving up and down?**" If the chest is moving up and down the problem is in the patient. If the chest is *not* moving up and down, the problem is in the equipment (anywhere from the ETT to the oxygen supply).

8.2.1.1 Chest Moving Up and Down (= Problem in the Patient)

Is there a pulse?

No – check rhythm and start CPR (rule out tension pneumothorax early).

Weak – i.e., hypotensive (rule out tension pneumothorax). Hypotension results in poor lung perfusion and increased ventilation/perfusion mismatch and a reduction in SpO_2 – give fluids ± adrenaline.

Normal – there is a *respiratory problem.*

Respiratory Problem

Check the peak airway pressure gauge on the ventilator and compare the reading to the reading before the problem. It will either have increased or be about the same.

Airway pressure increased:

Has the peak airway pressure on the ventilator increased since intubation?

If it has, is the chest movement symmetrical or asymmetrical?

Asymmetrical chest movement:

"Seesaw" = patient not paralyzed

One side moving/moving better:

- ETT in right main bronchus – pull back
- Tension pneumothorax – needle decompression
- Main bronchus plugged – suction catheter
- Large hemothorax – increase PEEP

If in doubt, get the self-inflating bag out and hand ventilate. This will give you more of a "feel" for the problem and larger tidal volumes can make asymmetrical chest movement more obvious.

Symmetrical chest movement:

- Lung contusions – increase PEEP
- Pulmonary edema – increase PEEP
- Bilateral secretions (unlikely) – suction catheter
- Bronchospasm (occurs immediately after intubation) – use i.v. ketamine for sedation

Airway pressure unchanged

The cause is usually worsening lung contusion/hematoma or pulmonary edema. All that can be done is to increase PEEP. If secretions are present in the ETT then clear with a suction catheter.

8.2.1.2 Chest *Not* Moving Up and Down (= Problem in the Equipment)

The problem lies somewhere between (and including) the ETT and the oxygen cylinder. Always start by looking at the

Pressure gauge on the ventilator. Is the pressure reading high and alarming (= obstruction/kinking) or is it reading low/not moving (= disconnection/ventilator failure)

Airway pressure high (>30 cm H_2O) (= occlusion)

Kinked: Ventilator tubing kinked somewhere, ETT kinked (possibly in the mouth) – pediatric ETTs are particularly prone to kinking as they are smaller and more compliant. This usually occurs outside the mouth.

(Severe bronchospasm may result in no chest movement, but this would occur immediately post induction/intubation. Periarrest tension pneumothorax may also result in no visible chest movement, but this should have been detected before getting to this stage.)

Airway pressure low (<10 cm H_2O) = disconnect/ventilator failure

If the needle on the ventilator is *completely* still, the ventilator has failed (i.e., the oxygen has run out for the majority of prehospital ventilators). Immediately change to a new cylinder, ensuring it has been turned on/the valve opened.

Disconnect:Check the ETT is not disconnected from the patient (i.e., extubated!). Look at the ETT length at the lips to see if it has moved out and look/feel for air/bubbles from the mouth.

If the ETT is secure, check for disconnections all the way from the ETT back along the catheter mount, HME and ventilator tubing to where the tubing connects to the ventilator.

If in doubt, get the self-inflating bag out and hand ventilate. Connect directly to the ETT and attach the oxygen tubing to another cylinder with a fir tree connector. This then takes all of the possible problems (other than the ETT) out of the equation.

8.2.2 Hypotension

Hypotension will be caused by one of four things:

1. Tension pneumothorax:Always rule this out before assuming blood loss/sedation is the cause. It should be recognized as a potential with chest injuries. The SpO_2 will be dropping and airway pressure increasing on the ventilator. Look for asymmetrical chest movement (one side moving more than the other).

2. Arrhythmia: This will be obvious from a quick glance at the ECG on the monitor. Treat as per ALS protocols.
3. Hypovolemia/anesthesia: This is the most likely cause but the Tension pneumothorax and arrhythmia should always be ruled out first. Treat with fluids ± ephedrine/adrenaline as indicated.
4. Pericardial tamponade: Consider this particularly after a penetrating wound to the left side of the thorax. Treatment is a clamshell thoracotomy, but this is only indicated during transfer if the patient loses their cardiac output altogether. Otherwise call ahead for surgical assistance in the emergency department.

References

Adnet F et al (1998) Pre-hospital intubation in the French system. Ann Emerg Med 32:454–459

Davis DP, Dunford JV et al (2004) The impact of hypoxia and hyperventilation on outcome after paramedic rapid sequence intubation of severely head injured patients. J Trauma 57:1–10

Easley RB, Segeleon JE, Haun SE, Tobias JD (2000) Prospective study of airway management of children requiring endotracheal intubation before admission to PICU. Crit Care Med 28:2058–2063

Helm M, Hauke J, Lampl LA (2002) prospective study of the quality of pre-hospital emergency ventilation in patients with severe head injury. BJA 88:345–349

Kluger MT, Short TG (1999) Aspiration during anaesthesia: a review from the Australian anesthetic incident monitoring study (AIMS). Anaesthesia 54:19–26

Norwood S, Myers MB, Butler TJ (1994) The safety of emergency neuromuscular blockade and orotracheal intubation in the acutely injured trauma patient. J Am Coll Surg 179:646–652

Reid C, Chan L, Tweeddale M (2004) The who, what and where of rapid sequence intubation. EMJ 21:296–301

Schwartz DE, Matthay MA, Cohen NH (1995) Death and other complications from emergency airway management in critically ill adults. Anaesthesiology 82:367–376

Sivilotti MLA, Ducharme J (1998) Randomised double-blind study on sedatives and haemodynamics during RSI in the emergency department: the SHRED study. Ann Emerg Med 31:313–324

Thomas CM (2004) Emergency tracheal intubation: complications associated with repeated laryngoscopic attempts. Anaes Anal 99:607–613

Appendices

Decision Making Algorithm for RSI

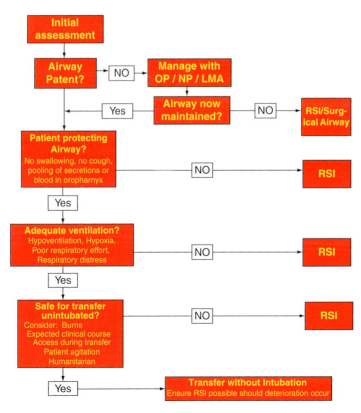

A. Griffiths et al., *Pre-Hospital Anaesthesia Handbook*,
DOI: 10.1007/978-1-84996-159-2_BM,
© Springer-Verlag London Limited 2010

Pre-RSI Checklist

GNAAS Pre-RSI Challenge-Response Check List

1. Pre-oxygenation	
Taking place and adequate oxygen available	Check
2. Preparation	
Baseline obs (SpO2, HR, BP, GCS, Pupils)	Check
Cannula	
Connected to fluid and runs easily	Check
Suction	
Working	Check
Back-up suction available	Check
Airway adjuncts (or escape ventilation)	
Guedel airway	Check
Two nasopharyngeal airways	Check
Ventilator and BVM connected to oxygen	Check
Emergency airways (LMA/Cricothyroidotomy)	Check
Tape or tie (Of appropriate length)	Check
Heat and moisture exchange filter (HMEF)	Check
Endotracheal tube	
Size chosen	Check
Cuff tested	Check
Drugs	
Induction agent dose chosen	Check
Suxamethonium dose chosen	Check
Drug giver briefed	Check
Angle piece or catheter mount	Check
Monitoring, including ECG, NIBP, SpO_2 $ETCO_2$	Check
Stethoscope	Check
Elastic bougie	Check
Laryngoscopes	
Two sizes chosen and working	Check
Syringe	
10 mL for cuff	Check
3. Premedication if required	Check
4. Paralysis and sedation	
In-line immobilizer briefed	Check
Cricoid pressure person briefed	Check
5. Passage of the tube $ETCO_2$?	Check
6. Post intubation management ABCDE	Check

Drug Dose and ETT Size Field Card

Field Card

Adrenaline	Dilution: 1 mL of 1:10,000 to 10 mL with saline Dose: 1–2 mL boluses titrated to response
Atropine	Dilution: 600 mcg (1 mL) up to 6 mL with saline (100 mcg/mL) (adult CPR dose 3 mg autojet) Dose: 10–20 mcg/kg pre-treatment/bradycardia
Atracurium	Dilution: Neat (10 mg/mL) in a 5 mL syringe Dose: 0.5 mg/kg (supplementary dose 0.15 mg/kg)
Ephedrine	Dilution: 1 mL (30 mg) up to 10 mL with saline (3 mg/mL) Dose: 1–2 mL (3–6 mg) titrated to response
Etomidate	Dilution: Neat (2 mg/mL) in a 10 mL syringe Dose: 0.2–0.3 mg/kg
Fentanyl	Dilution: Neat (50 mcg/mL) in 2 mL syringe Dose: 1–2 mcg/kg IV
Ketamine	Dilution: 200 mg up to 20 mL (10 mg/mL) with saline Dose: Analgesia 0.25–0.5 mg/kg IV (1–4 mg/kg IM) Anesthesia 1–2 mg/kg IV (5–10 mg/kg IM)
Midazolam	Dilution: 10 mg diluted to 10 mL (1 mg/mL) with saline Dose: 0.05–0.1 mg/kg initially (lower in elderly) 0.02 mg/kg maintenance bolus (1–2 mg)
Morphine	Dilution: 10 mg diluted to 10 mL (10 mg/mL) with saline (or with midazolam 10 mg/mL for sedation) Dose: 0.05–0.1 mg/kg initially 0.02 mg/kg maintenance bolus (1–2 mg)
Propofol	Dilution: 1% neat in a 50 mL syringe by infusion Dose: (Sedation) 1–4 mg/kg/h (15 mL/h start)
Suxamethonium	Dilution: Neat (50 mg/mL) 2 mL syringe (Peds-dilute) Dose: 1–1.5 mg/kg iv bolus
Pediatric weights	(Age + 4) × 2 kg (over 7 years age × 3 kg)
Endotracheal tube	Sizes: Male 8.0 mm, female 7.0 mm, children over 2 size = age/4 + 4.5 mm Lengths: Male 22–24 cm, female 20–22 cm, children over 2 years, age/2 + 12 cm

Failed Intubation Protocol

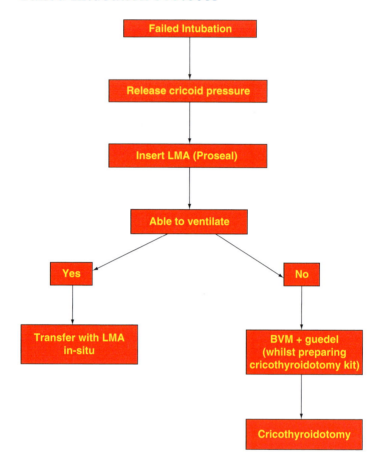

Actions on Desaturation

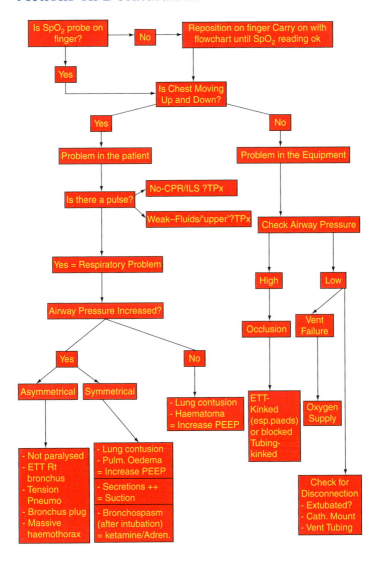

Emergency Cricothyroidotomy

Cricothyroidotomy is an emergency procedure and is usually performed when a secure airway needs to be achieved and attempts at orotracheal intubation have failed. It is contraindicated if other less radical means of securing the airway are feasible. There is the potential for significant complications, however, it may be a life-saving procedure and the prehospital medical team should be trained and prepared to undertake this if required.

The technique of surgical cricothyroidotomy we advocate is rapid, reliable and relatively easy. It addresses two problems that we have commonly seen in the pre-hospital environment which make some of the "standard" techniques less appropriate. These are bleeding from the incision and loss of the track into the airway before or during tube insertion (Fig. A.1). (The Difficult Airway Society now recommend a very similar technique.)

Indications

1. Failed airway by all other means.
2. Primary airway when other means not possible e.g., Severe facial trauma.

It is a rescue technique in most circumstances. Suitable equipment should be close at hand when it is anticipated that an airway will be particularly difficult. For example:

Airway trauma
Difficult anatomy
Burns to face and neck precluding jaw movement
Possible airway burns

In the cannot intubate/cannot ventilate situation, cricothyroidotomy is immediately indicated.

Anatomy

The cricothyroid membrane is identified by locating the laryngeal prominence (or notch) in the thyroid cartilage

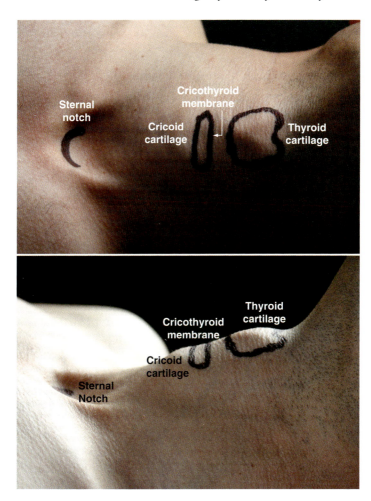

FIGURE A.1. The surface landmarks required to perform a cricothyroidotomy.

(Adams apple). One finger breath below in the midline is found the cricothyroid membrane. It is bounded inferiorly by the firm cricoid ring. This location is used as it is superficial and has less overlying thyroid and soft tissue than lower approaches. This leads to a lower incidence of significant bleeding.

Materials

1. Gloves.
2. Betadine solution to prepare the skin.
3. Swabs.
4. No. 11 scalpel blade.
5. Tracheal dilator.
6. Size 6 mm tracheostomy tube or size 6.0 mm cuffed endotracheal tube.
7. A 10 mL syringe for cuff inflation.
8. Bag valve mask (Ambu) connected to an oxygen source.
9. Securing tapes.

Technique (The Whole Procedure Should Only Take Around 30 s)

1. Prepare all necessary equipment and test the tracheostomy tube by inflating the cuff with 10 mL of air. Check it is intact and remains inflated after syringe removal.
2. Hyperextend the neck or use a neutral position if C spine injury is suspected.
3. Clean the skin with betadine solution.
4. Identify the cricothyroid membrane.
5. Anesthetise the skin over the membrane using the 10 mL syringe with 25-gauge needle with the 1% lignocaine if the patient is conscious.
6. Immobilize the larynx between thumb and forefinger of the left hand.
7. Make a 1.5 cm transverse incision of the skin over the cricothyroid membrane using a "stab/rocking" technique.
8. Leave the blade in position and push the tips of a tracheal dilator into the airway incision on either side of the blade and open it.
9. Remove the scalpel blade and insert a 6.5 mm cuffed tracheal tube into the hole held open by the dilators. The dilators may need to be rotated 90°.

10. Inflate the cuff and confirm tube position with $ETCO_2$ Monitoring. Ventilate via the usual catheter mount and HMEF if paralyzed and sedated. If alert with no respiratory failure, a standard variable flow oxygen mask may be placed over the tube having attached an HMEF to the tube (to prevent inhalation of dust, etc.).

11. Ensure endobronchial intubation has not taken place if using an orotracheal tube rather than a tracheal tube (consider cutting the tube shorter). Fix the tube securely in position with a tie or elastoplast. Do not tie the tape too tight around the neck.

12. Suction the trachea if required to clear blood post-procedure.

Use of the Laryngeal Mask Airway

Introduction

The LMA consists of three parts (Fig. A.2):

It provides an "oval seal around the laryngeal inlet" once the LMA is inserted and the cuff inflated. Once inserted, it lies at the junction of the digestive and respiratory tracts. The LMA has proven to be very effective in the management of airway crises.

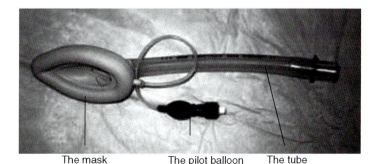

The mask   The pilot balloon   The tube

FIGURE A.2. A laryngeal mask airway.

Indications for the use of the LMA:

1. Failed intubation.
2. When ventilation with a BVM is required but not possible and PRSI is contraindicated (e.g., no trained team-member).

A standard LMA affords minimal protection to the trachea from gastric contents, however, can be quite effective at reducing contamination from upper airway bleeding. A Proseal™ LMA can provide a better seal and allow either free drainage or even suction of gastric contents through the gastric drainage port. It is therefore a better option if available.

Equipment for LMA Insertion

1. Appropriate size LMA.
2. Syringe with appropriate volume for LMA cuff inflation.
3. Water soluble lubricant.
4. Ventilation equipment (including $ETCO_2$).
5. Tape or other device(s) to secure LMA.

LMA size	Appropriate patient for use	Maximum cuff inflation volume (mL)
1	Under 5 kg	4
1.5	5–10 kg	7
2	10–20 kg	10
2.5	20–30 kg	14
3	Small adult	20
4	Adult	30
5	Large adult	40

Examination of the LMA Prior to Use

(a) Visually inspect the LMA cuff for tears or other abnormalities.
(b) Inspect the tube to ensure that it is free of blockage or loose particles.

(c) Deflate the cuff to ensure that it will maintain a vacuum.

(d) Inflate the cuff to ensure that it does not leak.

(e) Slowly deflate the cuff to form a smooth flat wedge shape that will pass easily around the back of the tongue and behind the epiglottis.

Lubrication of the LMA

(a) Use a water soluble lubricant to lubricate the LMA.

(b) Only lubricate the LMA just prior to insertion.

(c) Lubricate the back of the mask thoroughly.

NB: Avoid excessive amounts of lubricant on the anterior surface of the cuff or in the bowl of the mask. Inhalation of the lubricant following placement may result in coughing or obstruction.

Positioning of the Airway

Extend the head and flex the neck as for intubation (not with C-spine injury)

LMA Insertion Technique

1. Grasp the LMA by the tube, holding it like a pen as near as possible to the mask end. Place the tip of the LMA against the inner surface of the patient's upper teeth.

2. Under direct vision press the mask tip upwards against the hard palate to flatten it out. Advance the mask into the pharynx and ensure the tip remains flattened and avoids the tongue.

3. Keeping the neck flexed and head extended, press the mask into the posterior pharyngeal wall and continue to advance. This may be aided by an assistant pulling the lower jaw downwards. Visualize the posterior oral airway and ensure that the LMA is not folding over in the oral cavity as it is inserted. A jaw thrust or 45° rotation of the LMA may ease its passage over the tongue.

4. Continue insertion until the mask meets with resistance.
5. Inflate the mask with the recommended volume of air. Avoid over-inflating the LMA. Normally the mask should be allowed to rise up slightly out of the hypopharynx as it is inflated and finds its correct position.

Verify Placement of the LMA

1. Connect the LMA to a bag-valve mask device or low pressure ventilator.
2. Ventilate the patient while confirming equal breath sounds over both lungs in all fields and the absence of ventilatory sounds over the epigastrium.

Securing the LMA

1. A bite-block or roll of gauze may be used to prevent occlusion of the tube should the patient bite down.
2. The LMA can be secured using the same techniques as those employed to secure an endotracheal tube.

Trouble Shooting

1. Failure to press the deflated mask up against the hard palate and inadequate lubrication or deflation can cause the mask tip to fold back on itself.
2. Once the mask tip has started to fold over, this may progress, pushing the epiglottis into a down-folded position causing mechanical obstruction.
3. If in doubt, remove the LMA and repeat the process.

The Proseal LMA

It differs from the standard LMA as it has (Fig. A.3):

1. A gastric drainage tube that allows any liquid material to by-pass the larynx if regurgitation occurs.

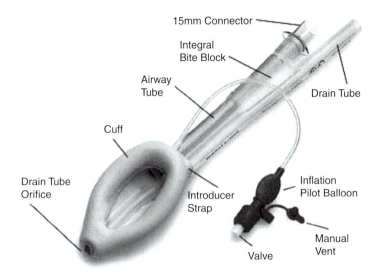

15mm Connector

Integral
Bite Block

Airway
Tube

Drain Tube

Cuff

Drain Tube
Orifice

Introducer
Strap

Inflation
Pilot Balloon

Manual
Vent

Valve

FIGURE A.3. A Proseal LMA. Reproduced by kind permission of
the Laryngeal Mack Company Ltd.

2. A posterior cuff that improves the airway seal. This
   may afford greater protection in the case of regurgitation
   and allow higher ventilatory pressures to be used (up to
   30 cm H_2O)

It should be used in preference to BVM (bag-valve-mask)
ventilation to prevent gastric inflation and therefore reduce
the risk of regurgitation and aspiration.

The Proseal™ LMA should be premounted on the metal
introducer. This stiffens the LMA and holds it in position during insertion. Without the introducer it can be very difficult to
insert in the manner of a standard LMA due to the flexible
reinforced airway tube.

An alternative method is to pass a bougie blindly into
the esophagus. The Proseal may then be inserted by passing the bougie through the drainage tube and railroading
the LMA into the oropharynx until it stops (when the tip
of the LMA reaches the esophageal inlet). When firmly
seated, the bougie should be removed and the cuff inflated.

Ventilation should then take place through the 15 mm connector.

It may rarely be inserted blindly into trapped patients in whom access is severely limited and augmentation of their ventilation is required.

Needle Thoracocentesis

This is a potentially life-saving maneuver in a casualty with suspected tension pneumothorax.

Procedure

1. Unless contraindicated (e.g., possible spinal injury), sit the casualty in an upright position (air rises).
2. Find the second intercostal space (ICS) in the midclavicular line. One method is to identify the manubriosternal junction (angle of Louis). In most people this is a bony prominence approximately 5 cm below the sternal notch adjacent to the second rib. The second ICS lies between the second and third ribs. In practice, because of the overlying muscles, the second ICS is the first easily definable space you come to on feeling down from the clavicle.
3. Attach a size 12 or 14G over-the-needle cannula to a 5 mL syringe. Fill with 1–2 mL of air. Insert through the skin and direct the needle just over the third rib. This should reduce the risk of haematoma and intercostal nerve damage. Use a two handed technique. Puncture the parietal pleura (this is usually <2 cm from the surface). Aspirate air to confirm the diagnosis (the plunger may be forced out by the high intrapleural pressure). Occasionally, tissue obstructs the cannula, so if no air is aspirated inject the 1–2 mL of air and aspirate again.
4. If the diagnosis is correct, advance the plastic cannula and withdraw the needle. An Ashermann seal can be placed over the cannula to stabilize the cannula, or secure with tape.

5. Cannulas can move slightly and no longer penetrate the pleura and hence cease to function very easily. Be prepared to insert another cannula if signs of tension pneumothorax recur.
6. If the patient is being transported awake, a chest drain must be inserted prior to transfer. If PRSI is being undertaken, a thoracostomy +/− chest drain must be performed immediately afterwards. Positive pressure ventilation can rapidly turn a pneumothorax into a tension pneumothorax or cause reaccumulation of a tension already relieved.

Thoracostomy ± Chest Drain Insertion

(The British military pre-packed, sterile set contains everything apart from LA.)

Fluid resuscitation and monitoring of vital signs must be in progress.

Equipment for a Chest Drain

Surgical scrub; sterile drapes and gloves.
20 mL syringe and needle.
Lignocaine 1% (20 mL).
Scalpel.
Blunt-nosed forceps.
Chest drainage kit including chest drain (= size 28), tubing and drainage bag with one-way valve (military pattern).
Suture material (e.g., No. 1 silk on a hand needle).
Zinc oxide tape.
Gauze swabs.
Scissors.
Dressing

Procedure

Thoracostomy

1. Determine the insertion site. The optimum position is in the fifth intercostal space just behind the anterior axillary line (i.e., just behind the lateral edge of pectoralis major muscle). This is approximately in line with the nipple in the male. Alternatively, count down from the second interspace, or estimate position from the lower border of the casualty's four fingers pressed hard in the axilla.
2. Clean the area with chlorhexidine/betadine (and drape ideally).
3. Anesthetise the skin, intercostal muscles and pleura.
4. Make a 2.5 cm incision through skin and subcutaneous tissue onto underlying muscle. Bluntly dissect apart the intercostal muscles using artery forceps.
5. Work over the top of the sixth rib to minimize damage to the neurovascular bundle.
6. Puncture the parietal pleura and insert a finger into the incision. Perform a 360° finger sweep to clear possible adhesions between lung and chest wall and exclude any herniated abdominal organs.
7. Check for bubbling air during transfer. Insert gloved finger to reopen if necessary.

Chest Drain Insertion

1. If not using the military pattern set, select the largest thoracostomy tube available (ideally >28F). Attach the tube to the drainage bag and advance the tube into the pleural space. Direct it anteriorly and upwards to the top of the thoracic cavity to relieve a pneumothorax (posteriorly for a haemothorax). Signs that you are in the correct place are bubbling around the tube as it is inserted and intermittent fogging of the chest tube during respiratory movements.
2. Insert the chest drain to a distance of 12–13 cm.

Complications of Chest Tube Insertion

Incorrect tube position inside or outside the chest cavity.

Laceration or puncture of intrathoracic or abdominal organs; this can be prevented by the finger sweep before inserting the chest tube.

Damage to the intercostal neurovascular bundle.

Local haematoma, haemothorax or intercostal neuritis/neuralgia.

Damage to the internal mammary artery if puncture site is too medial.

Dislodgement of the chest tube or disconnection from the drainage bag. Leaking drainage bag. Chest tube kinking or becoming blocked with blood clot.

Infection (e.g., local cellulitis, thoracic empyema).

Persistent pneumothorax from large primary defect; a second chest tube may be required.

Surgical emphysema (usually at tube site).

Mediastinal emphysema.

3. All the side holes must be well within the chest. Suture the tube in place using a mattress suture and Gibbon's flag or equivalent.
4. Apply a dressing and tape the tube to the chest.

Local Anesthetic Blocks

Femoral Nerve Block (Fascia Iliacus)

Indication: Analgesia for femoral shaft fractures allowing them to be reduced and splinted.
   Procedure:

1. Clean the skin.
2. Insert a blunted 18G needle just through the skin, 1 cm below the inguinal ligament (runs from anterior superior

iliac spine to pubic tubercle) at the junction of outer and middle third.
3. "Pop" through two distinct layers: Fascia lata then fascia iliacus
4. Aspirate the syringe before injecting to check the artery has not been punctured.
5. Inject 30–40 mL of a mixture of 1% lignocaine and 0.5% bupivicaine.

Onset: 5–15 min.
Duration: Up to 12 h.

Intercostal Nerve Blocks and Pleural Anesthesia

This technique is rarely used pre-hospital. It may be useful in older patients with fractured ribs when transfer times are long and the respiratory depressant effect of an opiate/opioid may be a problem.

Indication: Pain from fractured ribs to encourage adequate ventilation when patient breathing spontaneously. Alternative analgesia (e.g., fentanyl or ketamine) is more appropriate for most patients.

Complications: Pneumothorax – short, small gauge needles will reduce the risk.

Procedure

1. Palpate the rib to be blocked in the posterior axillary line. If the rib cannot be palpated – do not attempt the block.
2. Insert the needle through the skin until it hits bone close to the lower margin of the rib.
3. When the needle contacts bone, slowly move it downwards until it just slips under the lower margin of the rib.
4. Aspirate the syringe checking for absence of air and blood. Inject 5 mL of a mixture of 1% lignocaine and 0.5% bupiv-icaine. (Good analgesia will usually require additional blocks at one or two levels above and below the fracture(s).)

Index